Managing and Preventing Arthritis

MANAGING AND PREVENTING ARTHRITIS
The Natural Alternatives

George L. Redmon, N.D., Ph.D.

HOHM PRESS
Prescott, Arizona
1999

Cover design: Kim Johansen
Layout and design: Visual Perspectives, Phoenix, Arizona

Library of Congress Cataloging-in-Publication Data:
Redmon, George L., 1952-
    Managing and preventing arthritis : the natural alternatives /
George L. Redmon.
        p.   cm.
    Includes biographical references and index.
    ISBN 0-934252-90-4
    1. Arthritis--Alternative treatment.   2. Naturopathy.   I. Title.
RC933.R363   1999   98-45831
616.7'2206--dc21   CIP

HOHM PRESS
P.O. Box 2501
Prescott, AZ 86302
800-381-2700
http://www.hohmpress.com

Disclaimer: It is not the intent of the author to diagnose or prescribe, nor is it the purpose of this book to replace the services of a physician. The material is intended for educational purposes only. It is advisable to seek the services of a licensed, professional healthcare provider for any condition that may require medical or psychological services.

This book is dedicated to Della, whose physical struggle with a lifetime of pain, disease, discomfort and countless medical unpleasantries, inspired me to search for a better and more human way. Her courage, despite our misunderstanding concerning the progression and etiology of disease, finally made me realized that: Our greatest enemy is not the disease, it is our inability to realize our own individual innate potential to prevent or slow down its destructive forces.

Although gone in physical presence, she remains a powerful motivating force in my quest. May she rest in peace.

ACKNOWLEDGMENTS

The researcher is greatly indebted to Eric C. Dettrey and his secretarial support staff, especially Anita Anastasi, for the exceptional editorial and copy work done on this manuscript.

I also wish to express my deep and lasting appreciation to Pamela Peters, Ph.D., of The Center for Stress, Pain and Wellness Management, Wilmington, Delaware, for her support and guidance in the preparation of this book. I want to also thank Regina Sara Ryan and Rabia Tredeau of Hohm Press for providing the platform for this presentation's review and study.

CONTENTS

You have the ability to reverse the debilitating effects of arthritis. It is, however, very important to stop the process early.

Robert Willix, M.D.

Modern laboratory research on nutrients and cell chemistry suggest that most skeletal aging that occurs is not only preventable but reversible. Scientists are learning how to keep our muscular skeletal system strong and supple far longer than we ever thought possible. With the right care and attention you can expect to stay spry and active into your sixth, seventh and eighth decades of life.

Stuart M. Berger, M.D.

Although not in general use, knowledge of the cause of arthritis exists, as well as measures necessary for its prevention.

R.P. Walterson, M.D.

INTRODUCTION

In 1977, the Rockefeller Foundation, in conjunction with the Commission on Critical Choices for Americans, organized a group to study the problems of healthcare in the United States. John H. Knowles, M.D. headed this group of distinguished medical doctors. Walsh McDermott, M.D., in his report, "Evaluating the Physician and His Technology," stated that, "...with most microbial diseases, individual cases all tend to be alike, and the period from onset to full clinical illness is only a matter of days or hours." He went on to say that under these circumstances, the data supplied in the disease descriptions in textbooks is quite satisfactory. However, he maintained that the pattern of illness in the United States at that time was no longer mainly a matter of obvious microbial disease among the young, but one of highly diverse, hidden structural disease, frequently with several decades between actual (undetected) onset and outcome.

McDermott concluded that the technological evolution had shifted the disease pattern from the acute microbial toward the chronic non-microbial. Additionally, Dr. McDermott stated that this change had the paradoxical effect of appreciably reducing the physician's ability to forecast, and had created formidable problems in establishing the value of new therapies

THE EVIDENCE

The inability to forecast illness and its progression, and to evaluate correct therapies could be seen in the mounting incidence of the long-term degenerative nature of arthritis. According to statistics in 1977, some chronic disease afflicted 100 million Americans. According to the World Health Organization, in the United Kingdom, arthritis caused the loss of forty million workdays a year. Arthritis is Great Britain's most widespread disease, costing $300 million a year. In the United States, it had been estimated that one person in eleven suffered from this disease. Annual wage losses and medical costs totaled more than $3.5 billion annually. As a member of the Commission on Critical Choices for Americans, Dr. Thomas Lewis stated that over five million people in America had some form of rheumatoid arthritis or osteoarthritis. This was twenty years ago.

Today, figures have greatly increased. Based on current data, chronic degenerative diseases such as arthritis account for $425 billion in direct healthcare cost in the United States. Tack on the cost of medications, hospital visits and lost workdays, and those numbers escalate to about $659 billion. What is alarming about these dollar figures are the human statistical percentages they represent, as revealed by researchers at the University of California at San Francisco. For example, among individuals under the age of eighteen, at least twenty-five percent suffer from a chronic ailment, while current data estimates that thirty-three percent of the population aged 18-44 also has some form of chronic degenerative disorder. Those percentages increase to sixty-six percent for persons aged 45-64, and contrary to popular belief, the elderly account for only twenty-five percent of the population with chronic maladies, while those aged 18-64 comprise a whopping sixty percent.

FORECASTING THE FUTURE

Presently, forty million Americans have some form of arthritis. That number represents fifteen percent of the population, and recent studies show that these numbers will only increase. In fact, according to the Center for Disease Control and Prevention, by the year 2020 the number of Americans with arthritis will have increased by more than fifty-seven percent from today's numbers— the current forty million *could* escalate to over eighty million over the next two decades. This is alarming. The other disheartening factor is that researchers today know that there is a direct link between diet and the onset of the disease. Researchers also have determined that the most destructive aspect of the disease is uncontrolled free-radical aggression.

The investigation and validation of new therapies has become paramount, as conventional treatments in many cases seem to accelerate the degenerative nature of the disease. More and more people are seeking new innovative and non-invasive therapies geared toward disease prevention versus disease treatment. In fact, as cited by a major report entitled "Unconventional Medicine" (*New England Journal of Medicine*, 328; 246-52, 1993), researchers were astonished to find that sixty-one million Americans used some form of alternative or unconventional therapy in 1990 alone (the first year these statistics were available). According to this study, visits to alternative healthcare professionals totaled 425 million, as compared to 388 million visits to traditional medical doctors.

Additionally, as an exclamation to the above, a study released by the National Coalition on Health Care in Washington, D.C., revealed that seventy-nine percent of respondents felt that among healthcare providers, profit took precedence over consumer needs and safety.

Based on current trends and a move toward preventive healthcare, alternative or complementary health centers have sprouted up across the U.S. It has been estimated, based on studies conducted by the Health Policy Institute at the Medical College of Wisconsin in Milwaukee, that by the year 2010 the number of alternative medical clinics will increase by 124 percent over the current number in 1998. Also, recognizing these changing trends, in response to consumer request, the National Institutes of Health Office of Alternative Medicine (established in 1992) has allocated millions of dollars for research on how diets, plants, supplements and other natural-based modalities combat or counteract problems associated with the chronic degenerative diseases of today.

Furthermore, in response to recent proposals outlined by the Commission on Dietary Supplements, which was appointed by President Clinton in 1997, the USFDA (United States Food and Drug Administration) agreed with the commission that it should encourage continued research to assess the relationship between dietary supplements and the maintenance of health and/or the prevention of disease.

Current statistical changes in consumer health trends in the U.S. (Table i, below) provide an overview of the changing face of medicine.

Total number of plant-derived drugs prescribed by MDs.	120
Number of these drugs originally from folk medicine	90
US sales of herbs (1993, latest year available)	$1.13 billion
Annual growth in US herb sales	10-15%
Amount spent in US for MD care (1990)	$23.5 billion
Amount spent in US for complementary therapy (1990)	$13.7 billion
Amount spent in US for hospital care (1990)	$12.8 billion

Percentage of world population relying on traditional medicine	80%
Percentage of US adults who use complementary care	33%
Complementary care users who also visit MDs	83%

Table i.
Source: Catherine Fahey, "Medical Decisions," *The Energy Times*, Long Beach CA., 3:98: 49-53. Used with permission.

MY MOVE TOWARD ALTERNATIVE THERAPIES

Like most individuals, my move toward alternative therapies came in the aftermath of a serious illness and a recurring chronic problem. I fought and won the battle over Hodgkin's Disease—a form of cancer that attacks the lymphatic system. The lymphatic system can be described as a network that contains fluid armed with white blood cells that surround body cells. In essence, this fluid and its arsenal of white blood cells are directly involved with preserving the immune system. When this command post around our cells is compromised, as is the case with Hodgkin's Disease, our ability to defend against invading bacteria and other harmful toxins is severely diminished. Without proper treatment (usually radiation and chemotherapy), death can occur.

The experience of this disease changed my perception of myself, my lifestyle, my educational pursuits, and became my opportunity for the future. After weeks of conventional treatments, when no long- or short-term programs were put in place to enhance or re-build my immune system, I recognized that I would have to take responsibility for my own health. As a twenty-year-old undergraduate student in health, the onset of Hodgkin's Disease pointed me toward alternative and preventive healthcare.

MY ARTHRITIC NIGHTMARE

The second circumstance that drove my quest to learn as much as I could about alternative or preventive healthcare was an early bout with gout, a form of arthritis that attacks the joints. While researchers contend that gout may have some hereditary implications, it is caused by certain disruptions of proper metabolism. That is, with how the body breaks down and utilizes the food it consumes. In the person prone to gout attacks, incomplete protein digestion has been implicated in its onset. When protein digestion is incomplete, or because of over consumption, excess uric acid (a toxic by-product of protein digestion) can accumulate faster than it can be excreted. This causes the formation of crystals which usually end up in the joints (the knees, fingers, toes, ankles, etc.), causing severe pain and discomfort. Over time, repeated attacks can cause severe damage to joints and vital organs, especially the kidneys, as these crystallized deposits can interfere with their proper functioning.

As a twenty-year-old man, I was alarmed by the possibility of having to be fitted for an ankle brace and having to use a cane. The prospect of a lifetime of dependence upon medication was horrifying to me, although this was the prognosis of the foot and ankle specialists who were treating me at the time. Then, I was not quite aware of what was occurring and re-occurring within myself. Now, I know that there are a number of alternative protocols to eliminate the painful consequences of an attack of gout, as well as means to prevent one in the first place, which I discuss in this book.

The best thing about these holistic protocols is that they augment the actions of natural metabolic pathways instead of causing possible liver damage, kidney damage, hemolytic anemia, bone marrow depression, and kidney stones, as could Probenecid®, the medication I was prescribed. The most insidious of possible occurrences with the use of this proposed medication was the fact that acute attacks of gout could still occur after starting a daily regimen of use. Amazingly, I was not given this important piece of information by my personal physician at the time, or by any other medical professional.

For me, the biggest shock and concern was that there was no recommended plan of action in the aftermath of either Hodgkin's Disease or gout. No matter what the illness is, this should be everyone's major concern. Health does not exist in a vacuum. Health should flow ". . .from the way we live," says Dr. Andrew Weil, one of the country's top medical and alternative healthcare experts.

With this premise as a foundation, I hope you will continue to read on and learn how you can make a difference in how you feel. Recent research indicates that there are a number of nutritional supplements and other regimens that not only help to reduce the inflammation and pain associated with arthritis, but in some cases actually promote regression of the disease.

WHAT THIS BOOK COVERS

The focus of this book is to present a brief synopsis of the many viable options available in treating and preventing arthritic disturbances.

Chapter 1, "Understanding Arthritic Disturbances," presents a definition of arthritic disturbances, and then explains how they occur. It details the major types and specifies the causes of this disorder (free-radical destruction). Finally, it discusses why you may be at risk in resorting to the commonly prescribed NSAIDs (nonsteroidal anti-inflammatory drugs).

The purpose of Chapter 2, "The Antioxidant Necessity," is to clarify the destructive capabilities of uncontrolled free radicals, and to explain how antioxidants work to neutralize free-radical damage. The work of Dr. Denham Harman, the formulator of the "Free-Radical Theory of Aging" is discussed, as well as new product research on antioxidants.

Chapter 3, "Antioxidants That Fight Arthritis," focuses on current research in nutritional supplements and the role they play in alleviating arthritic disturbances. Studies conducted at the University of Missouri, research in England by Dr. Sheldon Hendler, and a synopsis of new research on individual antioxidants are covered in this chapter.

The intent of Chapter 4, "Natural Accessory Supplements," is to explore new and alternative therapies from a variety of sources and parts of the world. The theories and research on glycocyamine sulfate by Dr. William Lane, featured on the TV program *60 Minutes*, and author of *Sharks Don't Get Cancer* (1992) is cited. Studies conducted at the Queensland Medical Center in Australia concerning the efficacy of defensive toxins emitted by a marine animal known as the sea cucumber are also revealed.

Additionally, investigations by Dr. Karl Folkers with CoQ10 are discussed in Chapter 4, together with research conducted by Dr. Joel M. Kremer at the Albany Medical College in the Division of Rheumatology. Studies conducted on omega-3 fish oils by the Danish scientist John Dyerberg and Hans Olaf Bang are also presented.

Chapter 5, "Food is Your Best Medicine," explores food sensitivity and groups of foods that researchers have found beneficial to those suffering from the debilitating effects of arthritis. Foods that should be avoided by arthritic suffers are also listed. In addition, this chapter gives a brief overview of the concept of PH and its role in causing arthritic disturbances. The intent here is to show the reader how the diet affects the PH level, thereby affecting arthritis and a host of other maladies.

Chapter 6, "Alternatives in Managing Arthritis," is devoted to both past and present alternatives being used to lessen the severity of arthritic discomfort. Some topics or modalities covered are aromatherapy, homeopathy, mineral baths, detoxification, intestinal cleansing, acupuncture, acupressure, massage therapy, yoga, meditation and biofeedback. The overall goal of this chapter emphasizes that what Americans consider "alternative therapy" is not only accepted in most other parts of the world, but in many cases is the primary method of care.

The purpose of Chapter 7, "Getting the Help You Need," is to encourage motivation toward action. The reader is supplied with a list of organizations and practitioners of alternative healthcare. My goal here is to help the reader to set up and follow through with a formidable plan of action to minimize the debilitating effects of arthritis as well as to prevent its onset.

UNDERSTANDING ARTHRITIC DISTURBANCES

Arthritis is not a local disease of a particular joint, but
a systemic disorder which affects the whole body.

Paavo Airola, N.D.

Most people tend to regard arthritis as a single entity, a specific disease that has caused deterioration of a specific joint. However, this disease should be viewed as a disturbance of different organs and their correlated functions. In the absence of this view, the task of slowing down the progression of arthritis will not be attained. Max Warmbrand, N.D., an early pioneer of natural therapies states in *The Encyclopedia of Health and Nutrition* (1962):

When the close relationship between the general constitutional disorders and the arthritic manifestations is fully recognized, it becomes obvious that any approach that fails to eliminate or overcome the underlying causes of the disease is bound to fail in providing permanent results.

If we view arthritis as a disease caused by metabolic distur-bances, where does it originate from? Other pertinent questions that come to mind concerning this disease are:

1. What is arthritis?
2. Is its development a natural part of the aging process?
3. Is arthritis hereditary?
4. What causes the pain associated with its onset?
5. Are there different forms?
6. What treatments are available?
7. Is it curable?
   Let's begin to unravel some of the mystery of this disease.

და. და. და.

Arthritis results in inflammation and soreness of the joints. Re-search suggests that arthritis is related to the body's immune sys-tem. Either the body is unable to produce enough antibodies to prevent viruses from entering the joints, or antibodies that are pro-duced are unable to differentiate between viruses and healthy cells, thereby destroying the healthy cells. Arthritis may also result from an allergic reaction to certain foods.

The two main types of arthritis are osteoarthritis and rheuma-toid arthritis. Osteoarthritis develops as a result of the continuous wearing away of cartilage in a joint. Cartilage, which is a smooth, soft, pearly tissue, covers the ends of bones at the joints. It pro-vides a smooth surface for the bones to slide against, allowing easy movement of the joints. As a result of injury, or after years of use, cartilage becomes thin and may disappear. When enough has worn away, the rough surfaces of the bones rub together causing pain and stiffness. Osteoarthritis usually affects the weight-bearing joints, such as the hips and knees. Symptoms of osteoarthritis in-clude body stiffness and pain in the joints, especially during damp weather, in the morning, or after strenuous activity. Generally, inflammation of the joints does not accompany this disease. (See Figure 1.1.)

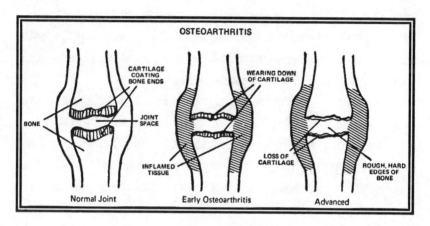

Figure 1.1
Nutrition Almanac. New York: McGraw Hill, 1990, p. 138.
Used with permission.

Osteoarthritis is the most common form of arthritis. It is esti-mated that by the year 2010 over seventy million people in the U.S. alone will have osteoarthritis. While the deterioration of this disease may show up as early as the age of twenty, in many cas-es, aside from injury or other possible predisposed medical or ge-netic reasons, osteoarthritis can take several decades (thirty or forty years) to develop. According to Dr. Michael T. Murray of Bastyr University, one of the country's leading naturopathic physi-cians and author of *Natural Alternatives to Over-the-Counter and Prescription Drugs* (1994, p. 66), eighty percent of all indi-viduals who suffer from osteoarthritis are over fifty. Dr. Murray al-so maintains that this malady is much more common in men un-der the age of forty-five, but seems to accelerate in women after age forty-five.

Although osteoarthritis is not considered as dangerous to vital organs as rheumatoid arthritis, it can be just as debilitating. Harris H. McILwain, M.D., a board-certified rheumatologist and gerontologist, and co-author of *Stop Osteo-Arthritis Now* (1996, pp. 12-14), insists that maintaining flexibility and strength is vital to preventing the limitations and immobility that osteoarthritis can cause. As we noted earlier, Dr. Stuart Berger (1984) asserts that ". . .with the right care you can expect to have good joint health into your sixth, seventh and eighth decades of life."

Rheumatoid arthritis, on the other hand, affects the entire body, not just one joint. Onset of this disease is often associated with physical or emotional stress. However, poor nutrition or bacterial infection may be just as likely a cause. Rheumatoid arthritis is generally considered to be much more serious than osteoarthritis. (See Figure 1.2).

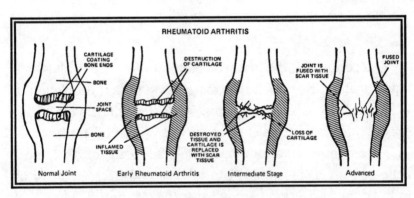

Figure 1.2
Source: *Nutrition Almanac.* New York: McGraw Hill, 1990, p. 138.
Used with permission.

Rheumatoid arthritis destroys the cartilage and tissues in and around the joints, and often the bone surfaces themselves. The body replaces the damaged tissue with scar tissue causing the spaces between the joints to become narrow and fuse together.

This causes the "stiffening" and "crippling" onset of the disease. Symptoms of rheumatoid arthritis include swelling and pain in the joints, fatigue, anemia, weight loss and fever. Many of these symptoms often disappear periodically, only to reappear at a later date.

THE QUESTION OF HEREDITY

There are currently over one hundred different known types of arthritis. According to David S. Pisetsky, M.D., Ph.D., a professor of medicine and assistant professor of immunology at Duke University Medical Center in Durham, North Carolina, there is no single diagnostic test that can determine if you have arthritis. He adds that, when trying to determine the type of arthritis you may have, questions concerning your genetic makeup and family history are critical to the overall diagnostic process (1991, p. 35). Researchers at the Arthritis Foundation, the organization founded in 1948, have found that certain people are predisposed toward arthritic disturbances due to traits passed in the genes from one generation to another (Kushner, 1984, p. 17).

IMMUNITY AND RHEUMATOID ARTHRITIS

Research has shown that arthritis can result from several different diseases, including bacterial infections and systemic lupus erythematous. These infections involve the production of free radicals by the immune system. Free radicals are highly reactive molecules that in times of stress can wreck havoc on cells, breaking down metabolic processes. Normally part of everyday metabolism, free radicals protect us from a host of environmental onslaughts—like smoke, fog, chemicals and stress, to name a few. However, these tiny molecules have been implicated as the causative factor for the acceleration of the aging process, and over sixty age-related degenerative diseases. (In the next chapter we will take a complete look at these highly destructive substances and their role in creating arthritic disturbances.)

Imagine the body at war with itself. That's what happens with rheumatoid arthritis. The body's own cells mistake body tissue for foreign substances. To repel the "invaders," the cells manufacture antibodies to attack the tissue. This is known as an auto-immune response. The body has sensed that there is some impending doom lurking and has initiated an all-out assault to render the foreign invader helpless. In this case, the assault causes much pain and discomfort for the arthritic individual since it contributes to damaging the cells in the joint membranes and degrading the joint lubricating fluids. While it affects fewer people—about seven million—than osteoarthritis, it attacks the whole body at once and is much more serious. However, by improving immune response with the right nutrients, rheumatoid arthritis can be prevented or regressed.

INVOKING THE AUTO-IMMUNE RESPONSE

The immune system is responsible for protecting us against pollens, allergens and all kinds of toxic substances. Billion of white blood cells patrol the immune system, and are biochemically ready to attack and destroy any foreign invaders.

Sensitivity to certain pollens and a host of other substances, including many foods, can trigger the onset of migraine headaches, nausea and dizziness. According to Alice S. Mills, M.D., a member of the American Academy of Allergy and the Department of Medicine at Northwestern University, the range of foods to which one may be allergic is almost without limit. In her book *Allergy: Facts and Fiction* (1983, p. 34), Dr. Mills states that "...the most common causes of these reactions are milk, grains (especially wheat), eggs, fish, shellfish, fruit (especially strawberries), nuts, chocolate, pork, pepper and mustard."

The problem for those suffering from arthritic disturbances centers on the fact that not only are white blood cells programmed to attack viruses, bacteria, cancer cells and other unidentified particles, they also attack and destroy any body tissue that is worn-out or run-down. Tissue that has been depressed due to injury, toxic build-up or abuse is subject to this attack, which is one of the major reasons why natural, alternative healthcare specialists recommend abstinence from animal protein. For example, eating a steak could pose several problems similar to smoking. Studies revealed that one pound of charcoal-broiled steak has as much benzopyrene (a cancer-causing agent) than the smoke of three hundred cigarettes (*Science* 145:53; 1964). Furthermore, when cooked meat is consumed, there is a proliferation of white blood cells found in the bloodstream. These manifestations all produce stress reactions, which cause the overproduction of free radicals. This, in turn, can trigger or "turn on" arthritis.

OTHER ARTHRITIC DISORDERS
GOUT

As previously discussed, gout is a form of arthritis that usually affects the joints, and can have a devastating effect on the proper functioning of the kidneys. According to Michael Murray, N.D. and Joseph Pizzorno, N.D. (1991) of Bastyr University in Seattle, Washington—the first joint of the big toe in many cases is involved in the first episode of an acute gout attack. The attacks usually occur at night, as a consequence of improper dietary considerations, trauma, injury, alcohol consumption, certain medications, as well as inadequate fluid intake.

Earl J. Brewer, M.D., founder and first chairman of the rheumatology section of the American Academy of Pediatrics, states that many interrelated events can trigger an acute episode of gout, including high blood pressure, stress, excessive alcohol consumption, obesity and rich foods, especially those loaded with purines—like organ meats and certain sea foods (1993).

Purines are essential to the transference of energy losses and gains that ensure proper functioning and reproduction of cells. However, they are also the basic substances of uric acid and are responsible for its formation in the body. Past and present research has clearly demonstrated that a reduction of foods that contain purines from the diet can have a positive effect in preventing the onset of an acute gout attack. In a nationwide arthritis survey conducted by consumer-oriented medical researchers Dana Sobel and Arthur C. Klein (authors of *Arthritis: What Works*, 1989, pp. 234-53), individuals suffering from rheumatoid arthritis, osteoarthritis and gout revealed that certain purine-rich foods triggered episodes of acute gout. By avoiding these foods, they were better able to control the formation of excess uric acid crystals. These foods and other food preferences are discussed in more detail in Chapter Five.

The Long Range Problems

The pain and discomfort associated with gout is caused by an internal metabolic defect in which excessive amounts of uric acid (a toxic by-product of protein breakdown) begin to accumulate in the system. The build-up of uric acid causes crystals to form, which further hinders its normal breakdown and elimination. When the eliminative organs become overwhelmed, there is, in essence, nowhere for the excess uric acid crystals to go. The surplus of crystals generally find its way to the joints, causing severe pain and discomfort.

With the advent of modern medicine and the plethora of drugs available today, current thinking concludes that gout is one of the easiest arthritic disorders to control, and that chronic acute gout attacks are rare. Many of these drugs, like Zyloprim® and Alloprin® are designed to inhibit the action of enzyme, xanthine oxidase, found in body tissues. By interfering with or inhibiting the action of this enzyme, these drugs can decrease the conversion of purines to uric acid. Other drugs, like colchicine and probenecid, are designed to slow down or eliminate inflammatory processes. However, these drugs actually block the proliferation of white blood cells at cites of inflammation. (This occurrence, as previously described, is part of the auto-immune response.) Lack of sufficient white blood cells will cause further pain, discomfort and deterioration of affected joints.

Furthermore, many of the drugs prescribed, such as Alloprin® (allopurinol) and colchicine, have mild-to-serious side effects, including liver and kidney damage, hair loss, nausea, abdominal cramping, headaches and dizziness. In fact, about ninety percent of those individuals who are predisposed to episodes of gout eventually suffer from some form of kidney malfunction, if not controlled (Petersdorf, 1983, pp. 517-528).

A General Misconception

Although gout is prevalent among adult men aged thirty and above, Branton Lachman, a professor of Pharmacy at the University of Southern California School of Pharmacy, reminds us that anyone can fall prey to this malady. This may be due in part to the fact that ten to twenty percent of the population suffers from or has problems associated with metabolic disturbances that encourage improper uric acid elimination.

Treatment Protocols for Gout
Conventional

As stated, conventional approaches employ a wide variety of medications to control the inflammatory process or to keep the formation of uric acid at normal levels. In addition, conventional protocol suggests that patients:

- Reduce alcohol consumption (alcohol inhibits the excretion of uric acid)
- Reduce weight
- Increase fluid intake, especially water
- Reduce fat in the diet
- Eliminate purine-rich foods.

Alternative

In naturopathic circles, the treatment protocol as outlined by conventional healthcare providers is also followed. The exception here, however, is an additional arsenal of naturally-occurring substances that can both alleviate or reduce the severity of acute gout attacks and elevated uric acid levels. An added plus there is that these substances do not cause damage to existing metabolic pathways and vital organs.

For example, the pharmacological attributes of the following nutritional and accessory supplements make them extremely useful in treatment of gout and other arthritic conditions:

1. *Cat's Claw* (Una DeGato)

This Peruvian herb—named Cat's Claw because of its claw-like thorns—has been used extensively as an anti-inflammatory agent, and for its ability to stimulate a strong immune response. Research has shown that Cat's Claw contains several naturally-occurring compounds called triter-pines, which have anti-inflammatory capabilities (*Journal of Natural Products,* 54 (2) (1991): 453-459).

2. *Devil's Claw* (Harpagophytum Procumbent)

This herb, used extensively in Africa and Europe, is best known for its ability to control pain and reduce inflammation. Tests in laboratories and clinics throughout Germany and France have shown that Devil's Claw's capabilities are comparable to cortisone and phenylbutazone—well-known anti-inflammatory drugs.

In addition, in numerous pharmacological trials, Devil's Claw has demonstrated the ability to reduce cholesterol and elevated uric acid levels.

3. *Charcoal*

Charcoal is known in alternative-medicine circles for its ability to relieve the build-up of gas in the system. Agatha Thrash, M.D., a pathologist, and co-founder of Uchee Pines Institute, a non-profit health-training institution in Seale, Alabama, uses charcoal to help reduce uric acid levels. She recommends taking 1/2 to 1 teaspoon, four times a day.

Alternative preventive measures for gout and for controlling uric acid levels also include the following:

- Consumption of red cherries between meals, which neutralizes uric acid
- Avoidance of salt, coffee, meat, eggs, fish, milk, alcohol and wheat products
- Focus on potassium-rich foods such as bananas and leafy green vegetables.

FIBROMYALGIA—THE DISTURBANCE OF THE DECADE

As we move into the next millennium, alternative healthcare researchers insist that current thinking must change concerning the existence of a form of arthritis that not only inflicts unrelenting pain, but also causes extreme emotional distress. This new form of arthritis is known as fibromyalgia, and has been classified as a syndrome.

The problem here, as with the more commonly known "chronic fatigue syndrome" (current data approximates that 2.4

million Americans suffer from this syndrome), is that in many cases patients show no clinical signs that anything is wrong. As a matter of fact, there is no known single cause of this syndrome. Additionally, there is no lab test to detect it, and subjects may show varying degrees of the symptoms associated with its onset and reoccurrence. As with the symptoms of chronic fatigue syndrome, which range from muscle fatigue, mental and emotion distress, severe joint pain without swelling, immune dysfunction and unrelenting fatigue, symptoms of fibromyalgia can disappear for years, only to reappear.

The problem for many medical professionals in identifying both chronic fatigue syndrome and fibromyalgia is the existence of an elusive plethora of symptoms. Because no two people react the same or exhibit the same symptoms all the time, the chronic fatigue syndrome has been called the "elusive entity." As such, for years many medical professionals doubted or dismissed these symptoms as being psychological in origin.

According to Ronald Hoffman, M.D., Director of the Hoffman Center for Holistic Medicine in New York City and one of the country's most renowned experts on chronic fatigue syndrome, there is no test "to prove" you have this disorder. As such, its diagnosis is done according to severity and time length of associated symptoms that restrict normal activity. Dr. Hoffman and associates maintain that the unfortunate error doctors often make when no clear-cut physiological reasons are present as the cause of a malady is to assume the condition to be psychologically based (1996, pp. 1473-1479).

Fibromyalgia also cannot be placed in any definitive category. The reason doctors may be unwilling to diagnose it is that, like chronic fatigue syndrome, no clinical test can confirm it. Hence its tag as a "syndrome" versus a disease. A disease, such as diabetes, can be defined as a condition that has a known origin. On the other hand, a syndrome is defined as a group of symptoms that together are characteristic of a specific disease. In other words, a syndrome is a collection of things or events all occurring at once. Fibromyalgia arthritic disturbances could be compared to the on-going events of a football game, hockey game, soccer game, a wrestling and a karate match all occurring at the same time, on the same playing field. For those who suffer from this malady, however, the game never ends.

Some common symptoms of fibromyalgia are:

- Aches and pains in the muscles, tendons and ligaments
- Fatigue and restlessness
- Muscle spasms
- Stiffness
- Headaches and paresthesia (tingly, prickly sensations)
- Sleep disorders
- Constant fatigue even after a restful night's sleep
- Depressed immune function.

Another Elusive Entity

The elusive pain associated with fibromyalgia is used to distinguish it somewhat from the chronic fatigue syndrome. Although no two individuals exhibit the same symptoms all the time or react the same to their negative effects, there are some similarities of symptoms. In fact, according to the American College of Rheumatology, the definite physical aspect associated with this disorder is the tenderness of at least eighteen different anatomical spots on the body. (See Figure 1.3.)

Fibromyalgia has been called a "wastebasket malady" due to the multitude of problems associated with it. Fibromyalgia patients, similar to victims of chronic fatigue syndrome, may suffer with associated symptoms one day and be full of energy the next. According to Earl Brewer, M.D., it is highly probable that twenty percent of the patients who visit an arthritis doctor have fibromyalgia,

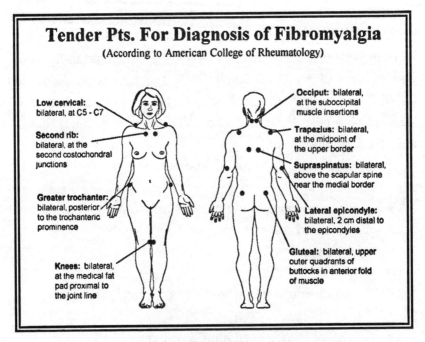

Figure 1.3
Source: Sahley, Billie Jay, Ph.D., *Malic Acid and Magnesium for Fibromyalgia and Chronic Pain Syndrome*. San Antonio, Texas, 1996, p.6

although not all doctors are able (or willing) to recognize it (1993). Hence, a fibromyalgia patient may be told that his or her painful symptoms are related to stress or depression. The other problem that doctors have to contend with in diagnosing fibromyalgia is that in many cases patients do not appear to be sick—some even report no signs of pain. (McIlwain, H.H., and D.F. Bruce, *The Fibromyalgia Handbook*. New York: Henry Holt, 1996, p. 159).

Incidence

Unlike gout, fibromyalgia disturbances are much more prevalent in middle-aged women, aged 25-55. Researchers put current female:male ratios at five to one. To put those ratios into proper perspective, it is estimated that today ten million Americans are afflicted with this arthritic disturbance.

Possible Causes

While researchers are still unsure exactly what causes fibromyalgia, individuals who suffer this and other forms of arthritis, including rheumatoid arthritis and lupus, may be predisposed toward its onset. Other possible causes of fibromyalgia are:

- Metabolic dysfunction
- Immune system disorder
- Allergic reactions to foods or yeast
- Viral or bacterial infections
- Prolonged stress
- Injury or illness
- Hereditary factors.

CONVENTIONAL TREATMENT—DANCING WITH DEATH

Having arthritis is like flying through a storm.
Once you are aboard, there is nothing you can do.
—paraphrase of Golda Meir

For the estimated forty million Americans who suffer from the debilitating effects of arthritis, Golda Meir's words accurately describe what dictates and dominates much of their daily existence. Many people think that the only way to cope with arthritic disturbances is to cover up or mask the symptoms of pain with medication. Julian Whitaker, M.D., founder and director of the Whitaker Wellness Institute in Newport Beach, California, and a noted medical practitioner who incorporates alternative medicine in his practice, asserts that the conventional drugs often prescribed by many doctors actually promote degradation of joints.

Nonsteroidal anti-inflammatory drugs (NSAIDs) such as as-pirin, ibuprofen (Motrin®), fenoprofen (Nalfon®) and indomethacin (Indocin®) may have the ability to alleviate the pain, swelling and inflammation associated with arthritic disturbances, but research has shown that these and other drugs in this category can also cause a variety of negative side effects. Gastrointestinal distress and bleeding, as well as headaches and dizziness have been linked to their use. One study showed that up to 2,600 people with rheumatoid arthritis die each year as a consequence of non-steroidal anti-inflammatory drugs, and 20,000 or more are hospi-talized each year for the negative side effects of these drugs. In general, the FDA attributes 10,000 to 20,000 deaths yearly to NSAIDs.

Other drugs, such as cortisone, which are meant to eliminate inflammatory changes in tissues, have been found to upset hor-monal balance with long-term secondary negative effects. In fact, cortisone can increase susceptibility to infections and peptic ul-cers, delay wound healing and over stimulate the adrenal glands, causing excessive fatigue.

Researchers also contend that these NSAIDs can cause "leaky-gut syndrome" (see Chapter Five). Dr. James Braly, author of *Food Allergy and Nutrition Revolution* (1992), reported that leaky-gut syndrome leads to allergic responses by the body, causing inflam-mation of the joints. More devastating is the fact that allergies to the deposited food particles (which leak from the gut) cause the body's immune system to attack the tissues around the joints, thereby leading to their destruction.

Another insidious result of using NSAIDs is that they also in-crease free-radical aggression. Researchers now known that meta-bolic imperfections can increase free-radical activity and play a ma-jor role in causing much of the related destruction and ill health as-sociated with arthritis. While many of the drugs prescribed may help relieve pain for the short term, they actually offer little hope toward correcting the underlying causes of the problem. This is clearly exhibited by the FDA's decision to remove the pain-reliever Duract® from the market. (Duract® is manufactured by Wyeth-Ayerst, the same drug company that had the popular diet drug Pondimine® (fenfluramine) and Redux® recalled.) This decision came in the wake of several deaths and at least eight individuals who required liver transplants after using Duract®. Although approved by the FDA, Duract® was not recommended for use beyond ten days because of its lethal capabilities. Despite strong warnings, doctors continued to prescribe this drug (up to 215 million prescriptions to date) to treat the symptoms associated with chronic arthritic disturbances. According to one industry analyst, it had been estimated that Duract® would generate $200-$250 million in new revenue for Wyeth-Ayerst.

In light of the massive amounts of revenue drug manufacturers generate, it is not hard to understand why special interest groups have attempted to place a stigma on alternative therapies, regardless of the fact that these natural remedies may be as effective and safer than their drug counterparts.

CONCLUSIONS

When we view the evolution of the problems associated with chronic arthritic disturbances, we can see a pattern that encourages the breakdown of metabolic pathways. As arthritis progresses, so do the etiologic manifestations of other metabolic disorders. That is, the pain and discomfort of arthritic disturbances have been related to other systematic dysfunctions. It is here that Dr. Max Warmbrand's remarks concerning the elimination of the underlying causes of the disease is crucial to finding long-term results, rather than simply focusing on pain relief.

Furthermore, as stated by Laura Aesoph, N.D., senior editor of *The Journal of Naturopathic Medicine* and author of *How to*

17

Eat Away Arthritis (1996), alternative measures may be better suited to attacking fibromyalgia and other arthritic disturbances due in part to the fact that the conceptual basis for natural modalities is oriented toward treating the whole individual, not just symptoms.

Let's move on to Chapter 2 and find out more about the real culprit responsible for causing such widespread arthritic disturbances.

THE ANTIOXIDANT NECESSITY

In the summer of 1991, scholars representing various sciences and social sciences from the United States, Europe and Australia met in symposium at the Harvard Club to discuss public health, lifestyle and the environment. This symposium, sponsored by the London-based Social Affairs Unit and New York's Manhattan Institute for Public Policy, was convened to ask and study: Why are the healthiest, longest-lived societies the world has ever seen, so concerned about their health?

According to this panel of distinguished scholars, there was little cause for believing that people from Western societies (namely the U.S.) were uniquely unhealthy. As stated by the panel:

> They appear instead to be the healthiest people who ever lived...No longer need they fear plague and famine. They are not infested with parasites. They are sound, their bodies strong. Almost invariably, they survive their infancy and overwhelmingly, their youth and middle age. The diseases that remain and kill, cancers and heart disease, are largely diseases of comparatively old age. Though they may be responsible for loss of lots of lives, they are not responsible for loss of many years of life (Berger, 1991).

Many past and present alternative healthcare providers, however, hold different views. As previously noted from the Commission on Critical Choices for Americans (1977), Dr. Walsh McDermott stated that, "The pattern of illness in the United States was no longer due to obvious microbial diseases, but highly diverse hidden structural disease."

Among many other distinguished researchers, the late Dr. Tom Spies, one of the most prominent health professionals in the U.S. during the 1950s and 60s, and a professor of nutrition and metabolism at Northwestern Medical School, had maintained that "germs" were no longer our principal enemy. According to Dr. Spies, our greatest emerging medical problem was what he considered to be a disturbance of the inner balance of the constituents of our tissues that are built from and maintained by necessary chemicals in the air we breath, the water we drink and the food we eat (Cheraskin et al., 1987, p. 7).

Furthermore, the famed medical and nutritional researchers Cheraskin, Ringsdorf and Clark, authors of *Diet and Disease*, note that although there has been a sharp decline in death and infectious disease rates, current data clearly shows a definite rise in chronic degenerative disorders, like arthritis, as well as in chronic pain and fatigue syndromes (1987, p. 39).

Many of these current disease patterns are causing a complete breakdown of natural metabolic processes that upset the body's attempt to maintain its own innate internal balance. The body may begin to attack itself in response to the build-up of toxins, causing severe pain and deterioration of joints, as well as rheumatic pain and discomfort.

The link between these diseases and the condition of our environment is unquestionable. According to Dr. Earl Mindell (1994, p. 24):

At no other time in history have the people of the world been so exposed to such a wide variety of pollutants in such high concentrations. We are bombarded with what scientists call xenobiotics—chemicals that are foreign to living organisms. If the body is healthy and functioning at its peak, it can generally detoxify and eliminate most of the pollutants without a great deal of damage.

Dr. Mindell's words are not encouraging to individuals who suffer from various types of arthritic disturbances. Due to the nature of this disorder, the metabolic pathways and eliminative organs tend to work overtime. In many cases, because chronic pain disorders begin to take their toll on various physiological systems that can cause severe toxemia, the arthritic patient's symptoms become more severe. The mishap of auto-immunity can occur as a direct result of a situation known as "emergency vicarious elimination," as well as by the continual psychological stress that often accompanies arthritis.

The term *emergency vicarious elimination* was coined by Henry C. Bieler, M.D., an early pioneer of nutritional medicine (1968, pp. 42-47). Dr. Bieler described it as an attempt by the body to use alternate channels of elimination when normal channels such as the kidneys, liver, lungs, skin and bowels are not functioning at peak capacity.

For example, the natural avenue of elimination for the liver is through the bowels, and the kidney's avenue is through the bladder and urethra. When these two natural avenues are clogged or overwhelmed with foreign toxins, or because of other metabolic malfunctions, poisonous by-products are released into the bloodstream. If these poisonous substances are not neutralized, not only can they damage tissue or serve as a precursor to arthritis, they can also accelerate aging and cause a host of chronic ailments.

Dr. Bieler maintains that when the middle layer of skin is forced into vicarious elimination, the diseases listed below can occur:

- Bursitis—inflammation of a bursa (a sac-like cavity usually found in or near joints)
- Encephalitis—inflammation of the brain
- Iritis—inflammation of the iris
- Meningitis—inflammation of the lining of the brain and spinal cord, with both mental and motor functions usually involved
- Neuritis—inflammation of the nerve
- Pericarditis—inflammation of the sac surrounding the heart
- Peritonitis—inflammation of the lining tissue of the abdominal cavity.

THE NUTRITIONAL CONNECTION

Could improper nutrition also play a role in exacerbating chronic degenerative states? Although the metabolic activity of many of our cells is still unknown, it is common knowledge that our cells get their supply of raw materials to do their work from circulating blood. The question then becomes: Do improper nutritional strategies inhibit the metabolic process due to their ability to encourage toxemia?

Despite the assertion just ten years ago by many prestigious organizations—such as the American Medical Association (AMA) and the Arthritis Foundation—that nutritional factors play a *minor* role in the causation of chronic arthritic disturbances, current thinking has definitely changed. Today, attention focuses on the understanding that proper nutrition or the lack of it is vital, not only to the maintenance of healthy joints, but to their construction. As expressed by the eminent nutritional researcher Dr. Roger J. Williams (author of *Nutrition Against Disease*, 1985, p. 44), ". . . we know that all the billions of cells in our bodies need a continuous supply of nutrients from nutritious food to extract and make the necessary materials which enable them (the cells) to perform their specialized functions."

In the absence of these nutrients from circulating blood, what happens to the metabolic machinery? Just as plants will feed on and utilize toxic elements in the soil or water when proper nutrients are in short supply, cells in the human body will operate in much the same fashion. Mounting evidence suggests that if cells do not get the optimal amounts of the nutritional materials they need, cell functions are compromised. Improper nutrition, coupled with the rise in the use of over-the-counter medications as well as prescribed drugs, have encouraged the evolution of arthritic disturbances into chronic syndromes. Besides exhibiting episodes of chronic pain and unrelenting fatigue, these distur- bances are multi-functional—with both negative physiological and psychological manifestations.

Alternative therapists contend that the old paradigm that sug- gests that aging is a major factor in the onset of these chronic pain syndromes is incorrect. In 1985, Carlton Fredericks, Ph.D., in his book, *Arthritis: Don't Learn To Live With It,* argued that the concept of aging as an excuse for a degenerative disease is based on correlation, meaning that aging and these disorders go hand in hand. However, according to Fredericks, "correlation" never proves "causation," though it may imply it (p. 26).

EXAMINING CELLULAR DAMAGE

Dr. Richard Passwater, Ph.D., a well-known nutritional and biological researcher, director of research at Solgar Nutrition Re- search Center in Berlin, Maryland, states that cellular aging starts before birth and is a major factor in the aging process of all bio- logical and physiological systems. Passwater asserts that, in actu- ality, destruction or cellular aging is altered or hastened not by the passing of time, but by improper chemical reactions. On this premise, he insists that if we could find a way to control or neutralize these circumventive reactions, we would be able to slow down, reverse or better control the progression of many of the so-called age-related degenerative disorders, such as arthritis (1985).

The internal human environment, like everything in nature, has a check and balance system to maintain health. It is imperative that optimal chemical or cellular balance occurs. The human body is not a fixed entity in structure or function. (It has no 100,000-mile warranty.) Many inherent physiological as well as self-imposed and outside influences can contribute to cellular degeneration.

Andrew Weil, M.D., one of today's most notable medical and alternative healthcare practitioners maintains that each human body has one or more weak points, and that it is important to know those points, especially because they are the places that tend to register stress as early warning signs of any impending breakdown of health. Dr. Weil says that, "If you learn to recognize these signals, this will help you notice patterns of developing problems in its subtle stages, which will ultimately improve your chances of correcting the problem" (*Health and Healing*, p. 60).

One common negative signal in the onset, progression and subsequent regression of arthritis is the presence or absence of free radicals—highly reactive molecules, which have the capability of causing much destruction and the interruption of common metabolic activities. In fact, these substances have been implicated as the cause of arthritis and at least sixty age-related disorders. Furthermore, the onset and duration of the symptoms of arthritis proliferates the production of free radicals.

THE MAJOR CAUSE OF ARTHRITIS

Dr. Sherry Rogers, author of *Wellness Against All Odds* (1992, p. 27), maintains that classically there has been no known cause and no effective treatment for osteoarthritis. Yet, Dr. Robert D. Willix, who developed the only open-heart-surgery program in the state of South Dakota, believed otherwise. He decided to end his career as a famous (and wealthy) surgeon because he felt that surgery was the extreme end to the degeneration of chronic structural diseases. According to Dr. Willix, who now runs a preventive medical clinic in Florida, scientists have found out that a single cause is responsible for aging, as well as for cancer, heart disease, stroke and arthritis. That single agent is the free radical. Dr. Willix maintains that the actions of antioxidants and their ability to combat the debilitating effects of free radicals, is the most important medical discovery in the last fifty years.

WHAT ARE FREE RADICALS?

Free radicals are chemically reactive molecules. Unlike a stable molecule in which every atom is ringed by pairs of electrons, the free radical carries an unmatched electron with a strong impulse to mate. By snatching an electron from a neighbor, it can set off a chain reaction that wreaks widespread havoc on cells, eating away at their membranes and damaging their genetic material. The damage that free radicals do in the body is known as oxidation (which is why the substances that neutralize and slow down this damage have been named *antioxidants*). Mindell states (1994):

> We can think of oxidation as similar to what happens to metal when it rusts, or an apple when it turns brown. Unstable oxygen molecules go to war in the body, grabbing onto other cells in their attempt to become stable. In the process, they damage cells including the genetic coding, or the DNA in the cells. Once the process of oxidation

begins, it can be hard to stop, and the consequences range from heart disease and high blood pressure to arthritis and birth defects.

The body has to handle free radicals every day. In fact, they are necessary. Free radicals are products of normal metabolism in cells; they help generate energy within the cell. They are also responsible for producing melanin pigment, which must be present in order for the formation of images. Free radicals are involved with the process of photosynthesis—they work on the green pigment known as chlorophyll to facilitate the exchange of oxygen and carbon dioxide that make up our atmosphere. Unfortunately, however, free radicals are everywhere. They are created by exercise, by exposure to sunlight, x-rays, ozone, tobacco smoke, car exhaust and other environmental pollutants. Moreover, as we age, the numbers of free radicals increase in the body, and as they do, the chances also increase that these cellular saboteurs can do great harm.

Free radicals can trigger inflammation and cause damage to blood vessels. They attack cellular membranes, damaging them with sometimes drastic results. For example, lysosomes (particles found in the cytoplasm of cells) contain powerful enzymes (acid hydolases) that break down tissue constituents. When lysomal membranes are ruptured by free radicals, these enzymes are released, causing damage to surrounding tissues. Rheumatoid arthritis is an example of this type of attack.

While we have built-in enzyme systems to help protect and sustain the cells from the onslaught of free radicals, this control system has imperfections, and can become overwhelmed. Without naturally-occurring enzymes like superoxide dismutase (SOD for short) and glutathione peroxidase, we would be unable to survive. Pearson and Shaw (1982) remind us that all air-breathing life on our planet has had to evolve with these enzymes intact in order to subsist.

Additional Problems with Free Radicals

According to the free-radical theory formulated by Dr. Denham Harman in the 1950s, the random and irreversible reactions ignited by these molecules produce a multiplicity of detrimental reactions. The five basic types of damage caused by free radicals are:

1. Lipid Fat Peroxidation:
    During this process, free radicals start to work on fat compounds in the body, causing them to turn rancid, thus releasing more free radicals.

2. Cross-linking:
    This mishap causes proteins and DNA to fuse together, much like coils in a mattress. When this occurs, pain, stiffness, and decreased mobility of joints may result, while collagen—your connective tissue—can lose its elasticity and flexibility.

3. Membrane Damage:
    When the cellular membrane is in good condition, it serves as a control mechanism, allowing food and nutrients into the cell, while expelling waste. Free-radical damage to cell membranes has been cited as a major causative factor, or precursor, which allows auto-immune diseases, arthritic disturbances and a host of other negative disease states to flourish.

4. Lysosome Damage:
    Uncontrolled free-radical aggression can have a devastating effect on cell membranes or lysosomes—cellular structures that contain enzymes that are responsible for breaking down waste and foreign matter. When held in the cell in small sacs, these enzymes sacs are beneficial to cellular health and metabolism. It is when these sacs rupture or become weakened that the cell begins to literally digest itself, leading to pain and other related symptoms that precede

metabolic dysfunction. Free radicals have been implicated as a major cause of lysosomal damage to cells.

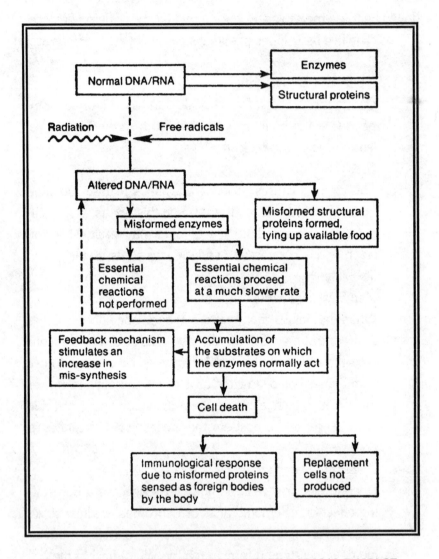

Figure 2.1 - **THE PROGRESSION OF FREE-RADICAL DAMAGE**
Source: Dr. Richard Passwater, *Selenium As Food and Medicine.*
New Canaan, Connecticut: Keats Publishing, 1980, p. 224.
Used with permission.

5. Lipofuscin:

Lipofuscin is an accumulation of age pigments that can inhibit cellular communication functions. It is speculated that these yellowish-brown or brown spots that appear in and on the skin but are not freckles, birthmarks or scars, clog up brain cells. Researchers also believe that these age- or liver spots (as they are sometimes called) are leftover waste material that the lysosome enzymes are unable to destroy. Current data suggests that when this pigment begins to accumulate at levels of up to seventy percent of cellular volume, neurons die. According to biochemical researchers Pearson and Shaw (1982), this pigment accumulates at the apex of the nerve cell, blocking the flow of vital nutrients to the other nerve fibers extending from the apex. Eventually these nerve fibers die, followed by the death of the cell, and thus ending cellular communication.

In retrospect, the destruction that free radicals cause is the biological equivalent to a terrorist bomber gone berserk in the control room of a nuclear reactor. The cumulative levels of oxidation caused by free radicals can put millions, even billions of cells out of commission.

Now that scientists have confirmed that free-radical aggression can accelerate the body's decline of live active cells, the question then becomes how can we neutralize the destructive effects of these necessary but deadly substances.

THE MIGHTY ANTIOXIDANTS

Just like the early wonder drugs, antibiotics and penicillin which eradicated the problems of the killer infectious diseases, antioxidants can prevent killer diseases and help al-

leviate the symptoms and side effects of inflammatory disorders such as arthritis.

—Dr. Richard Passwater (1995, p. 20)

In the past, arthritis and its crippling effects were thought to
have no cure, and no known action to stop or slow their process.
Treatment often involved using steroids and synthetic drugs to
reduce the pain and swelling. According to Robert H. Davis,
Ph.D., a professor in the Department of Physiology at the Pennsylvania College of Pediatric Medicine, these drugs can cause side
effects that are sometimes worse than the cure. Today, however,
as cited by Dr. Earl Mindell, author of *What You Should Know
About the Super Antioxidant Miracle* (1996), we know that antioxidants have a profound influence on diseases of the connective
tissue, such as arthritis. Current data has confirmed that antioxidants can play a major role in reducing the pain of arthritis and
can greatly reduce the need for medications such as aspirin or
acetaminophen.

Dr. Mindell's reports are corroborated by investigation by European investigators Lassen and Horder, who have found that individuals who supplemented their diet with the antioxidant selenium had much healthier joints than those using a placebo. There is
corroborative evidence that a deficiency of selenium may accelerate damage to weakened joints. Therefore, it is suggested that selenium may play a vital role in treating rheumatoid arthritis (*Scandinavian Journal of Rheumatology*, 14 [April-June]: 97-101;
1985). However, health officials maintain that supplementation of
selenium should not exceed 200 mcgs. daily.

Mindell (1994, p. 11) calls his top-four antioxidants *the aces*:
vitamin A (beta carotene), vitamin C, vitamin E and selenium. He
cites a study by M.S. Menkes published in the *New England Journal of Medicine* showing that these four "aces" significantly re-

duced the risk of lung cancer, even in people who smoked cigarettes (Mindell, 1994, p. 27).

Willix (1994) notes two studies presented in 1992 at the American Heart Association's 65th Scientific Session. The first study involved almost 90,000 women. Those who took vitamin E for more than two years cut their risk of heart disease almost in half compared to those who did not. The second study involved 45,720 middle-aged and elderly men. Those who had taken vitamin E for more than two years had a twenty-six percent lower risk of heart disease.

In addition to the above studies, doctors at the Harvard Medical School after a ten-year, 22,000-male-physician study, found some astonishing results. Men who were given 50 mg. of beta-carotene every other day suffered half as many heart attacks and deaths as those taking the placebos. Harvard researchers have begun trials in 45,000 post-menopausal women to see if similar effects occur (cited in Lieberman, 1997, p. 66).

The antioxidant vitamin C, one of the most well-known vitamins for many years, had been advocated by the late Linus Pauling, the eminent chemist and Nobel Prize winner. The late Dr. Pauling, a ninety-one-year-old author, lecturer and scientific researcher, felt that the optimum intake of vitamin C that gave people the best protection against free radicals was perhaps one hundred times the current RDA. He suggested that vitamin C should be taken every day, six grams to eighteen grams (6,000 to 18,000 milligrams), or more. From an extensive review of medical and scientific literature, Dr. Pauling concluded that vitamin C also combats a number of viral disorders: hepatitis, measles and mumps, viral pneumonia, herpes labial (fever blisters), certain types of meningitis, influenza, and the common cold. According to Pauling, vitamin C seems to exert both a preventive and a therapeutic effect when taken in optimum amounts.

Current research indicates that diets high in the antioxidants found in fresh fruits, and green-leafy vegetables may reduce the risks associated with free-radical damage. Researchers also suggest supplementing the diet with vitamin C, vitamin E, and beta carotene. Clinical studies show that drugs prescribed for arthritis significantly lower blood and tissue levels of vitamin C.

Vitamin C is responsible for the building of collagen, the protein factor that keeps tissues firm and well-knit. When collagen is strong and the tissues firmly held together, they can stop an infection from further invasion, whether it is a bacteria, a virus, or an allergy such as hay fever.

New Product Research on Antioxidants

Researchers continue to investigate the amazing benefits of antioxidants. While vitamin C, vitamin E and beta-carotene are probably the most well known, there are, however, others such as:

- Superoxide Dismutase—commonly known as SOD. Super-dioxide Dismutase is a group of natural enzymes made in the body. They can prevent damage to the synovial fluid and membranes. SOD is used extensively in racehorse training to alleviate the joint inflammations of thoroughbreds. The injectable version of bovine copper zinc SOD (known as orgotein) has been reported to be useful in some cases of rheumatoid arthritis.

- Pantothenic Acid (Calcium Pantothenate)—a member of the vitamin B family. Nearly fifty years ago, Nelson and co-workers noted that young rats acutely deficient in pantothenic acid suffered defects in growth and development of bone and cartilage (*Proceedings of the Society for Experimental Biology and Medicine*, 73:31, 1950). The defects were reversed with pantothenate supplementation. In another study, Barton, Wright and Elliot (*Lancet*, 2:862, 1963) reported that blood levels of pantothenic acid are significantly lower in humans with rheumatoid arthritis than in normal individuals. Furthermore, the General Practitioner Group conducted a double-blind study (*Practitioner*, 224:208, 1980) that recorded "highly significant effects for oral calcium pantothenate in reducing the duration of morning stiffness, degree of disability, and severity of pain in subjects suffering from rheumatoid arthritis."

In addition, Shari Lieberman, Ph.D., a well-known certified nutritional specialist and a professor at the University of Bridgeport School of Human Nutrition, has found that some arthritic individuals have lower levels of pantothenic acid than non-arthritics; the lower the levels, the more severe the painful symptoms of arthritis tend to be. Dr. Lieberman states in her book, *The Real Vitamin and Mineral Book*, (1996, p. 114-5), " . . .the supplementation of pantothenic acid (vitamin B5) . . . has had dramatic results in reducing the general symptoms of morning stiffness, disability and pain."

Dr. Lieberman suggests using the following dose ranges when administering or introducing pantothenic acid as a viable option in reducing the negative effects of arthritis:

- Joint Inflammation: 100-2,000 mg. daily
- Lupus: 6 grams daily, while gradually reducing the range to 2-4 grams daily for maintenance as negative symptoms begin to disappear or subside.
- Osteo- and Rheumatoid Arthritis: 50 to 2,000 mg. daily.

Also, Gary Null, Ph.D. (1998), the host of the nationally syndicated radio program "Natural Living with Gary Null," a respected alternative practitioner, states that pantothenic acid is vital to a strong immune response and is critical to maintaining good joint health. This is due, in part, to pantothenic acid's role as a building block for cortisone. According to Dr. Null, without the cortisone the body naturally produces, everyone would invariably suffer from arthritic disturbances (1998, p.29).

- Pycnogenol®—a natural substance used widely in Europe because of its value as an antioxidant. Extracted from the bark of pine trees (Pinus Pinaster), Pycnogenol® has a molecular structure similar to compounds found in the family of flavonoids—known to have powerful antioxidant properties. Bioflavonoids, which enhance the action of vitamin C, are a subgroup of flavonoids. Research conducted by scientists at Horphag Overseas Limited in France have shown that proanthocyanadin, the substance found in pine bark, is what makes Pyncogenol® such a powerful antioxidant, and twenty times more effective than vitamin C. Research indicates that Pycnogenol® has strong anti-inflammatory capabilities.

Additional Benefits of Antioxidants

Like most nutrients in nature, antioxidants have multiple attributes and are found in abundance from many different sources. Harry Demopoulous, M.D., a well-known antioxidant and anti-aging researcher states that, the role of ". . .antioxidants in combating free radical aggression is as important of a discovery as was Pasteur's germ theory of disease." (Kronhausen,1989)

In addition to fighting free radicals, Dr. Robert Willix claims that antioxidants help alleviate or prevent the harmful effects of a host of other diseases besides arthritis, heart disease and cancer. As evidence he cited the following:

- a Harvard study that showed that taking vitamin E long-term (more than two years) can cut your risk of heart attacks almost in half, and

- a report in *The Journal of the National Cancer Institute* that showed similar results for a study of 29,584 people in China, aged forty to sixty-nine.

The Chinese rates of esophageal and stomach cancer are among the highest in the world, more than ten times the U.S. rate. In this study, those who took a daily dose of beta carotene, vitamin E and selenium suffered nine percent fewer deaths than those who didn't (Willix, 1994, pp. 8-10).

Researchers in Paris found that topical application of antioxidants (C,E, and beta carotene) greatly reduced the long-term destruction to the skin caused by the ultraviolet radiation of sunlight (discussed in, *The Philadelphia Daily News*, 8-24-98, p. 23).

In conclusion, Dr. Denham Harman, who first formulated the free-radical theory of aging in 1956, has suggested three methods of experimentally reducing free-radical damage in the bodies of experimental animals:

1. Reduce calories in the diet to reduce the production of free radicals in metabolism.
2. Minimize dietary components such as copper and polyunsaturated fats which tend to increase free-radical production.
3. Add to the diet one or more free-radical quenchers, such as vitamin E, C, A, B-1, B-5, B-6, zinc, selenium and cysteine.

THE FINAL CONNECTION

The late Dr. Carlton Fredericks in his masterpiece, *Arthritis: Don't Learn To Live With It* (1985), strongly reminds the arthritic patient that there is one major omission in orthodox treatments for arthritis. This overlooked factor is YOU, the individual, and your failure to take responsibility for your sickness, but more importantly for your recovery. If your outlook or attitude falls short here, Dr. Fredericks vehemently protests against falling prey to a false sense of security and dependency, in which you complacently swallow an unending series of pills prescribed by a series of physicians; pills that in reality only address the pain and associated discomfort of arthritis.

You are without a doubt the final connection here, and play a major role in the success of the outcome of your alternative path. This train of thought today is an extension of that of the early pioneers of alternative medicine. Moving with this train, and realizing that you are the most important variable in this process, will strengthen your resolve and thus promote the use of preventive measures versus treatment. As Dr. Fredericks stated (1985, p. 16):

> Only when the patient begins to participate in seeking and exploring all the possible roads to help and recovery will treatment be effective, rather than a masking of symptoms.

ANTIOXIDANTS THAT FIGHT ARTHRITIS

Recent studies have linked several natural substances that have shown remarkable effects against
the pain and inflammation associated with arthritis.

Steven Schechter, N.D.

With population studies showing that we are living longer, and
with the corresponding rise in the number of individuals
who have or will develop arthritic symptoms, "joint health" has become a major topic. New studies have confirmed the efficacy of a
number of natural supplements that are as effective as their pharmaceutical counterparts, without the long-term negative side effects. In this chapter we will:

1. Review new research on antioxidants and their use in treating
   and preventing arthritic disturbances.
2. Examine a number of nutritional supplements that have shown
   great benefits in alleviating the volatile patterns of arthritis.
3. Take a look at how you can determine your very own "individual antioxidant profile."

NEW ANTIOXIDANT RESEARCH
THE POWER OF BIOFLAVONOIDS

Bioflavonoids are found in abundance in nature, in the pulp rinds of citrus fruits such as oranges, lemons and limes. They are also part of the pigments that give fruits and vegetables their bright colors. Once known as vitamin P, bioflavonoids (named by the famed physician and Nobel Prize winner, Albert Szent-Gyorgyi, the discover of vitamin C) were initially known for their ability to enhance the utilization of vitamin C. Bioflavonoids were also extensively researched and used because of their ability to preserve capillary integrity.

Current research has uncovered some interesting facts concerning the antioxidant capabilities of bioflavonoids. Known in alternative circles as "nature's newest heroes," they have been found to be twenty times more potent in antioxidant capacity than vitamin C, and fifty times more effective than vitamin E as free-radical scavengers. Ongoing trials concerning the effectiveness of bioflavonoids continue to date.

Much of the early research done in France with extracts of Pinus Maritima pine bark and grape seeds have led to the classification of a group of bioflavonoids known as *Oligomeric Proanthocyanidin*, OPCs for short. These compounds are currently considered to be the most powerful antioxidants in existence.

Because of its ability to protect vitamin C from oxidation and enhance its synthesis, bioflavonoids protect valuable collagen. Bioflavonoid OPCs have the unique ability of not only being able to neutralize free-radical aggression, but of actually inhibiting the formation of free radicals.

Some of the benefits OPCs present to the individual who is prone to arthritic dysfunction are their ability to:

1. Boost the immune response
2. Control the release of histamine

3. Improve circulation
4. Increase flexibility of joints
5. Increase energy
6. Promote healing
7. Increase strength of cartilage, ligaments and tendons
8. Act as an anti-aging nutrient
9. Inhibit cross-linking (which leads to acceleration of the aging process and is characterized by the hardening of the joints, fluid loss in the joints, rigidity of the arteries)
10. Recycle vitamin C and vitamin E for use.

The Need To Supplement

Since the human body is incapable of producing its own supply of OPCs (bioflavonoids), many natural-heathcare providers (myself included) strongly recommend supplementation. There is no current RDA (recommended daily allowance) for bioflavonoids. However, the suggested intake for general health is 150 to 300 milligrams a day. For optimum dosages that take into account individual biochemistry, need, and overall health, Shari Lieberman, M.A., R.D., a well-known clinical nutritionist, recommends that 500 to 5000 mg. of bioflavonoids be taken by adult men and women with equal amounts of vitamin C. As noted in the previous chapter, in her clinical experience, Lieberman has found the following dose ranges of bioflavonoids to be most effective. For inflamed joints: 3,000-10,000 mg.; for capillary damage: 500-5,000 mg.

Special Note: Due to wide latitude and high dosages as cited above, supplementation at these levels should only been done under the guidance of a healthcare professional.

CAROTENOIDS

Carotenoids are the compounds found in fruits and vegetables that give them their orange, yellow, red, and green colors. Over the last decade, hundreds of clinical trials have examined the antioxidant capabilities of beta-carotene. Although beta-carotene is without a doubt one of the best known of the carotenoids, to date researchers have identified over five hundred different carotenoids, many of which have stronger antioxidant activity than beta-carotene.

Recently, renewed interest has grown in the use of carotenoids (also called carotenes) as viable adjuncts to help manage arthritic disturbances, due in part to new research that suggests that carotenoid concentration in tissues may be a key factor in determining life span. Also known as "pro vitamin A," carotenoids have strong staying power, and as such, influence tissue health to a great degree.

Laboratory and epidemiological studies (which compares data from one country or region within a country to one another) have demonstrated that antioxidants work synergistically. This has prompted health officials to recommend taking supplements or consuming foods rich in many different carotenoids. Furthermore, there is evidence that carotenes inhibit or diminish leukotriene production (leukotrienes are responsible for provoking inflammatory responses to allergens, and are 1,000 times more destructive than histamine, a common inflammatory substance).

There is no current recommended dose range for carotenoids. The U.S. Department of Agriculture and the prestigious National Cancer Institute, however, recommend diets that provide 5 to 6 mg. of these antioxidants a day. The Alliance for Aging Research recommends 10 to 30 mg. daily. Carotenoid supplements can be purchased in local health food and vitamin stores.

DHEA

DHEA (dehydroepiandrosterone) is a hormone that is produced in the body from cholesterol. It is the most abundant hormone found in the body. C. Norman Shealy, M.D., Ph.D., the originator of "Transcutaneous Electrical Nerve Stimulation" (TENS), the first biofeedback training program for chronic pain, and the founding president of the American Holistic Medical Association, states that "...research has demonstrated that DHEA may be the most critical single chemical in the body predicting disease or health" (1996, p. 5).

DHEA levels appear to decline with advancing age. One of the most important functions of DHEA is that of helping the body adapt to stress caused by the over stimulation of the adrenal glands in response to an impending stressor, such as arthritic discomfort. When this happens, the hormones glucocorticoids (or cortisol) are pumped into the bloodstream by the adrenal glands, naturally helping the body tolerate pain. A synthetic version used by the medical profession is injected into arthritic joints.

Cortisol is part of a family of steroidal drugs, which are carbon copies of the hormones made by the body. These hormones—dexamethasone, hydrocortisone or cortisol, and prednisone—are widely prescribed under the trade names: Decadron®, Cortef® and Deltasone®. While these drugs may offer temporary relief, they can also have serious side effects. These steroidal drugs can cause:

- depression
- eye damage
- stomach cramping
- diarrhea

- diabetes
- psychological problems
- ulcers
- increased susceptibility to infection

Relief of pain in afflicted joints from these cortisol (steroids) hormones can last for sometimes three to six months. In the process, however, your body's natural production of these hormones may stop. Since the most important function of these natural hormones is to modulate the body's ability to adapt to physical stress, such as trauma to weakened joints, you may be compromising the long-term health of affected joints.

Dr. Shealy states that, "...studies (in animals) have shown that DHEA plays a major role in adjusting glucocorticoids levels in times of physical stress" (1996, p. 6). Arthur C. Guyton, M.D., who has served as Chairman of the Department of Physiology and Biophysics at the University of Mississippi School of Medicine maintains that in the absence of these natural glucocorticoids, metabolic pathways become deranged and despondent. Such despondency prevents the body from being able to protect itself from any chronic condition that may cause inflammation or complete destruction of tissues (1969, p. 421).

DHEA And Cartilage

Recent clinical trials in DHEA's ability to reduce the pain, swelling and stiffness associated with arthritis have revealed why it is a viable alternative to synthetic hormones. DHEA accelerates the production of IGF-1: insulin growth factor. IGF-1 has the ability to enhance proteoglycan synthesis. Proteoglycan synthesis is related to the natural production of connective tissue.

DHEA also plays a role in countering the negative effects that interleukin-1 has on cartilage. Interleukin-1 is a substance produced by your immune system that helps destroy toxins and other foreign invaders that can compromise the body's ability to stay healthy. However, it emits a substance that seems to hasten the breakdown of valuable cartilage. DHEA is instrumental in neutralizing this occurrence.

Special Note: DHEA can be purchased as a nutritional supplement in health food and drug stores without a prescription. Dose ranges are usually 10 to 50 mg. Follow the manufacturer's suggested usage. DHEA shouldn't be used by any individual with a family history of breast, ovarian or prostate cancer. Please check with your healthcare professional before implementing DHEA into your overall regimen.

GLUTATHIONE

Glutathione—known as GSH or glutathione peroxidase—is manufactured by the body and is part of a very powerful internal enzyme system that can be compared to an elite special forces team whose job is to neutralize hostile agents. In this case, the enemy target would be potentially harmful free radicals.

Although glutathione naturally occurs in the body, it may be wise to incorporate this antioxidant as part of your daily regimen. The eminent antioxidant researchers Kronhausen, Kronhausen and Demopoulous (1989) assert that without its inborn presence, or due to low levels, some individuals (especially the aged) do not respond well to inflammatory reactions. Without adequate GSH, prostaglandin production may be severely compromised. (Prostaglandins are a group of hormone-like substances that have a controlling effect on inflammatory response, contraction of smooth muscles and dilation of blood vessels, thus promoting good circulation.)

Additionally, because GSH may assist in enhancing prostaglandin activity, data suggest that glutathione plays a major part in stimulating and attracting leukocytes—agents which eat up bacteria, viruses or other harmful compounds that may ignite an inflammatory response or suddenly cause a acute arthritic attack.

Glutathione (an amino acid protein) is comprised of three different amino acid proteins—glycine, glutamic acid and cysteine. Evidence indicates that glutathione levels in the body can be heightened by the use of the three aforementioned amino acids. Also, maintaining adequate levels of GSH are dependent on vitamin E and the mineral, selenium.

Earl Mindell (author of *What You Should Know About The Super Antioxidant Miracle*) reminds us that GSH levels diminish as we get older and that their dynamic functional capabilities become seriously impaired. Dr. Mindell maintains that, to add insult to injury, this antioxidant's ability to minimize the effects of reoccurring arthritic episodes is hampered by the use of pharmaceutical drugs that stress the liver—such as acetaminophen (Tylenol®) and aspirin, birth control pills and hormone replacement therapy.

Studies done in England have shown a direct correlation between low glutathione levels (in the elderly) and an increase in arthritis, diabetes and other chronic diseases.

GREEN TEA

For thousands of years the Chinese have used herbal teas as a means to fight mild depression, promote relaxation, boost resistance and energy. Today, new research indicates that green tea is the second most frequently consumed drink (water being first) in the world. The reason for the growing popularity of this tea (already used extensively in Asia) is due to recent research out of the National Cancer Institute, Columbia University, The Medical College of Ohio in Toledo, and the University of Texas Center for Alternative Medicine. Scientists have discovered that green tea naturally contains potent immune stimulants that contain anti-bacterial and anti-cancer chemicals. Green tea also has powerful antioxidant capabilities. The substances responsible for the health-giving benefits of green tea are known as polyphenols. The class of polyphenols found in green tea are catechins and flavonoids that exhibit extraordinary antioxidant capabilities. Extensive research focuses on green tea's most abundant polyphenol—epigallocatechin gallate (EGCG)—which, according to current data, inhibits the production of the enzyme urokinase, which is partially responsible for cancer cell growth and migration.

Many alternative practitioners recommend consumption of green tea due to its overall health benefits. However, due to rich contents of flavonoids (a special type of bioflavonoid), green tea may also be very beneficial in preventing arthritic malfunctions and controlling allergic reactions. Additionally, because green tea also exhibits strong thermogenic abilities it has the capacity to assist the body in burning off calories and producing energy. This process would help reduce unhealthy weight or maintain healthy weight levels, thus cutting down additional stress to weakened joints. Green tea also promotes healthy circulation, which is one of the most problematic disturbances for the arthritic individual.

Four Cups A Day

Due to its caffeine content, green tea consumption should be done in moderation. A cup of green tea contains about 35-50 mg. of caffeine in contrast to 75-95 mg. in a cup of coffee. Besides containing polyphenols, green tea is also rich in carotenoids and chlorophyll, revered for its ability to supply energy to tired cells as well as its ability to help cleanse and fortify sluggish organs.

There is one other important reason to consider substituting green tea in place of certain other drinks. According to Patrick Quillin, Ph.D., R.D. (1987, pp. 307-321), some researchers speculate that arthritis is aggravated by consumption of cold fluids with meals, while hot herbal teas may facilitate the absorption of essential fatty acids. Essential fatty acids like evening oil of primrose, gamma linolenic acid (GLA), EPA and DHA (omega-3 fish oils) have potent anti-inflammatory actions, as well as help to keep joints lubricated. The reasoning behind this theory, as cited by Dr. Quillin, is the fact that cold fluids change the surface tension of fats in the intestines, thus inhibiting proper assimilation of essential fatty acids. These fats are extremely beneficial to the arthritic individual and cannot be made by the body.

Current research indicates that one to four cups of green tea is an adequate daily amount.

ISOFLAVONES

Isoflavones belong to a growing number of naturally-occurring plant substances that are called phytochemicals. Phytochemicals are the biologically active compounds that have medical properties found in specific plants. These compounds give plants their colors, odor and flavor, and are also responsible for protecting plants against harmful pathogens. Current research suggests that these compounds may offer the same protection to humans. Isoflavones, found in soybeans, have been extensively researched for their ability to minimize the negative effects of menopause and to fight cancer (especially hormonally-related cancers, such as breast cancer). Investigations concerning the benefits of isoflavones were prompted by research that indicated that Asian and Japanese diets rich in soy were responsible for a lower incidence of breast cancer and a number of other chronic disorders.

Research at the National Cancer Institute, Harvard University and the University of Alabama have shown that soy isoflavones and their phytochemicals have powerful antioxidant properties.

According to Dr. Earl Mindell (*Earl Mindell's Soy Miracle*, 1995), soy foods come naturally packaged with a strong antioxidant and chelating agent—phytic acid. A chelating agent has the ability to facilitate the use and elimination of minerals, thus inhibiting them from finding their way into weakened joints and lodging into tissues.

Based on his research, Mindell found that phytic acid has a strong attraction to iron. When oxygen is present, iron will create free radicals, possibly causing arthritic disturbances. Isoflavones can block the production of free radicals because of its phytic acid content. The phytic acid actually binds with iron to prevent its oxidation.

The soybean is one of the most nutritious foods you can consume. Acccording to Mindell in *The Joy of Soy* (pp. 67-69), it is easy to incorporate soy foods into a daily diet. He suggests consuming 100 to 160 grams (which equals about 4-8 ounces) of varied soy products a day. (To get more information on soy products, recipes and current research, call 1-800-825-5769 to get a free copy of the *U.S. Soy Foods Directory.*)

The following information represents the approximate isoflavone content of some popular soy foods:

Soy Milk (1/2 cup) ....40 mg.
Tofu (1/2 cup)..................40 mg.
Tempeh (1/2 cup)............40 mg.
Miso (1/2 cup) ....40 mg.
Textured Soy Protein
 (1/2 cup cooked) ....35 mg.
Soy Flour (1/2 cup)..........50 mg.
Soy Beans (1/2 cup) ....35 mg.
Soy Nuts (1oz.) ....40 mg.

U. S. Soy Foods Directory, Indianapolis, Ind., 1998, p.9.

The Big Three

Investigations into the efficacy of soy have revealed that three isoflavones are responsible for its rejuvenating abilities. These are genistein, paidzein and glyciten. Research has indicated that these isoflavones can:

- Inhibit bone degradation
- Prevent osteoporosis
- Stimulate antioxidant activity
- Reduce the pain and inflammation associated with arthritis
- Lower cholesterol
- Be used as an adjunct to or as a viable hormone replacement therapy option (consult your health professional)
- Enhance the immune response
- Control angiogenesis aggression—the formation of new blood vessels as a result of some pathogen.

Research into the phenomenon of angiogenesis has increased due to the efforts of Dr. William Lane. In his book *Sharks Don't Get Cancer* (1992), Dr. Lane details his experiments with shark cartilage. According to Dr. Lane, sharks do not contract cancer, nor do they develop arthritis or many chronic conditions associated with aging. Numerous clinical trials have shown that shark cartilage prohibits angiogenesis.

Isoflavonoids inhibit angiogenesis. According to Derrick M. DeSilva, Jr., M.D. of the Raritan Bay Medical Center in Perth Amboy, New Jersey, and president of the American Nutraceutical Association, the formation of new blood vessels (angiogenesis) rarely occurs in healthy adults. In fact, as stated by Dr. DeSilva, normal angiogenesis can be pathological and can promote certain diseases such as:

- Cancer
- Psoriasis
- Rheumatoid arthritis
- Diabetic retinopathy
- Macular degeneration (loss of eyesight).

Angiogenesis and Rheumatoid Arthritis

During chronic arthritic attacks, weakened and damaged joints speed up the production of angiogenic substances in the synovial space of the joints. It is within these spaces that the synovial fluid resides. The synovial fluid provides the material that keeps the joints lubricated, much like the oil that lubricates the cylinders in your car. This reduces the friction, and lessens the wear and tear and associated pain. Alternative healthcare practitioners today recommend supplementing the diet with numerous types of soy products that are rich in isoflavones. Andrew Weil, M.D. (author of *Eight Weeks To Optimum Health,* 1997) states that:

In my opinion, one of the healthiest dietary changes people can make is to substitute soy foods for some (or all) of the animal foods they now eat. (p.70)

Today, over fifty percent of the world's production of soy products occurs in the U.S. Soy products and their isoflavonoid compounds come in the form of:

- Soybeans
- Soy burgers
- Soy cheeses
- Soy flour
- Soy granules
- Soy hot dogs
- Soy milk
- Soy isoflavonoid supplements
- Soy sausages

When purchasing soy products, I recommend that you stay away from products labelled "isolated soy," as they are processed and may not contain naturally-occurring isoflavones, especially the big three isoflavones—genistein, daidzein and glyciten. Instead, I strongly recommend the consumption of a generous supply and variety of organic on soy products, supplemented by isoflavonoid tablets or capsules. Tablets should be standardized for isoflavonoid content. This means that the raw materials used to make them (via special processing techniques) have a certain percentage of the biologically active components of the proposed supplement, in this case isoflavonoids.

Stephen L. DeFelice, M.D., Chairman of the Foundation for Innovation in Medicine in Cranford, N.J., supports these recommendations. Although epidemiological studies show that certain foods prevent disease, many phytochemicals—like isoflavones—are not always found in therapeutic doses in food alone.

Special Note: For some individuals soy products are contraindicated due to allergic responses to them. Please refer to Chapter 6,

"Food Is Your Best Medicine," for guidelines to test your sensitivity to various foods.

LIPOIC ACID

Over the last several years lipoic acid has gained national attention, in part because of its ability to act as both a fat- and water-soluble nutrient. The problem with many antioxidants is that because of their solubility their activity is limited to either inside or outside the cell. However, due to the findings of Dr. Lester Packer of the University of California at Berkeley, a pioneer in lipoic acid research, and others, we now know that lipoic acid is a universal antioxidant. This means that it has the ability to work both inside and outside the cell environment. One of the most exciting aspects of lipoic acid is that it can regenerate the activity of other antioxidants like vitamins C and E, thus enhancing and strengthening their overall capability. When these powerful antioxidants neutralize the harmful effects of free radicals, they are used up in the process. Lipoic acid has the ability to jump start (so to speak) the power of these antioxidants as their capacity in neutralizing the harmful effects of free radicals begins to fade, much like jump-starting a dead car battery. This is part of the reason that lipoic acid is known as a "metabolic enhancer." Lipoic acid, therefore, would be of great benefit to the individual who is prone to arthritic disturbance and increased free-radical aggression.

Lipoic acid exhibits its strong antioxidant capabilities inside the cell, especially within those structures called the mitochondria, where food is converted into the energy that fuels metabolic processes. Metabolic processes (or metabolism) can be defined as all the actions that are anabolic (like building new bone, tissues or cartilage) and catabolic (like the destruction of bone, tissue or cartilage) within the body. While the cycles of anabolism and catabolism occur endlessly, any sound health-building program should be centered on minimizing catabolic cycles.

Lipoic acid is also intimately involved with a metabolic process known as glycolysis, which is the first step in converting blood sugar to energy. This process enables the body to better utilize glucose, providing needed energy to the system to help offset the debilitating effects of arthritis. There is also evidence that lipoic acid actually enhances the entry of glucose (the energy molecule) into muscle cells versus fat cells. Lipoic acid may help reduce muscle fatigue and protect red blood cells from oxidation, while neutralizing the destructive nature of free radicals.

Morton Walker, D.P.M., a well-known medical journalist, suggests that lipoic acid is an essential nutrient. This assumption is based on the fact that lipoic acid needs to be present to facilitate the action of other substances. Since arthritis is a result of and can be classified as a multi-dysfunctional disorder, meaning that the pain and discomfort associated with it are expressions of many different problems, lipoic acid would be of great benefit in its treatment. Because of its diverse antioxidant capabilities, I strongly recommend its use.

Current data suggests that taking 100 mg. of lipoic acid three times daily will help minimize cellular damage.

QUERCETIN

Bioflavonoids naturally contain anti-inflammatory agents that help modulate the pain and swelling associated with arthritis. One bioflavonoid that is gaining wide acceptance and use is quercetin. Quercetin has the ability to slow down or inhibit the release of histamine. When allergens enter the system, histamines are released that cause allergic reactions to invading allergens. Symptoms range from red, itchy eyes, sneezing, sinus blockage and congestion, coughing and running nose to possible arthritic disturbances.

The conventional protocol for dealing with these symptoms is the use of a class of drugs known as antihistamines. These drugs stop the release of histamine by locking onto cellular receptor sites.

This action could be compared to placing duct tape over your light switch to prevent its use. Quercetin, rather than binding to these sites, naturally impedes or suppresses histamine formation, as well as other substances that can ignite arthritic flare-ups. One such substance that querectin suppresses is leukotrienes.

Within the immune system, leukotrienes are related to white blood cells. Recent research has shown that leukotrienes have powerful destructive capabilities as they relate to arthritic disorders. For example, leukotrienes can cause severe broncho-constriction, including extensive damage to the lungs. This can undermine the arthritic individual's ability to defend against allergens and auto-immune responses. Leukotrienes are 1,000 times stronger in their ability to cause inflammation than histamine.

One of the most effective ways to counteract the negative effects of histamine and allergic responses to allergens is with quercetin. C. Leigh Broadhurst, Ph.D., a practicing allergist and a nutritional consultant, advises his patients to supplement their diets with at least 1,000 mg. daily when an allergic reaction occurs. Julian Whitaker, M.D., suggests taking 250 to 500 mg. daily, five to ten minutes after meals.

Special Note: Because quercetin needs to be absorbed properly, Michael T. Murray, N.D. (1994) states that quercetin should be taken between meals along with bromelin (a digestive enzyme found in pineapples) to facilitate its absorption.

ANTIOXIDANT SUPPLEMENTS THAT FIGHT ARTHRITIS

In our discussion thus far we have taken a look at research on a number of antioxidants that have a positive effect on arthritic disturbances. Although not commonly used in a program to manage the debilitating aspects of arthritis, several nutritional supplements can also provide support. In the next segment of this chapter we shall review a few of these supplements. Besides providing support, many of these nutritional supplements have antioxidant capabilities of their own.

VITAMIN B-1

This vitamin helps prevent cross-linking, the abnormal bonding and stiffening of collagen and elastin, the "protein glue" in the white fibers of our tendons, bones, cartilage, skin and all other connective tissue. By counteracting this bonding of our tissues, B-1 helps keep us youthfully flexible, provided we start taking it early enough in life. Michael T. Murray, N.D. (*Seven Valuable Tips for Managing Osteoarthritis*, 1998), asserts that osteoarthritis is more prevalent in men under the age of forty-five and after age forty-five in women. Incorporating the use of this supplement may be much more beneficial by taking it as a twenty-year-old, than when symptoms first begin.

VITAMIN B-3

This vitamin, also known as niacin, nicotinic acid, niacinamide and inositol hexanicotinate (all interchangeable terms) is classified as a "vasodilator," a substance that assists in widening arteries, thus promoting proper blood flow. When the arteries narrow, this encourages blood clotting and cholesterol buildup. This hampers circulation, which in turn can cause hardening of the arteries and increase the likelihood of initiating arthritic disturbances.

Early research by Dr. William Kaufman (1949) had demonstrated niacin's ability to diminish the pain associated with arthritis. The amazing results of a number of case histories were outlined in Dr. Kaufman's book, *The Common Form of Joint Dysfunction: Its Incidence and Treatment*, and reintroduced by the nutritional researchers Adams and Murray (1978), whose past and present essays on the medical applications of nutrition are well known. For example, a thirty-nine-year-old female who suffered from mild arthritic discomfort, low back pain and reoccurring joint stiffness was given 150 milligrams of niacin every three hours for six doses daily. Within one month, Dr. Kauffman had reported considerable improvement in the patient's range of movement and discomfort.

According to Adams and Murray, Dr. Kaufman had reported additional benefits form his patients who were administered niacin (in its niacinamide form). These benefits included:

- Improved digestion
- Increased energy
- Enhanced mental clarity
- Improved muscle strength.

Unfortunately, this early research went unnoticed by most conventional doctors, and was overshadowed by a new steroidal hormone substance that had become the therapy of choice. That substance was cortisone.

Although Dr. Kaufman's early research never received its due, continued research into niacin's efficacy has turned up some astonishing findings. Due to relentless efforts of present day scientists like Hoffer and Walker (authors of *Ortho-Molecular Nutrition*, 1978) niacin is used to treat and prevent a number of metabolic disorders such as:

- Clinical depression
- Schizophrenia
- Psychopathic disorders
- Elevated cholesterol levels
- Chronic fatigue
- Attention deficit disorder
- Migraine headaches
- Impotency

Researchers have discovered that niacin is intimately involved with more than fifty metabolic reactions in the body. Niacin is also crucial to proper nervous system function; and in cases of deficiency, severe pain in extremities, headaches, sleep disruption and energy losses can occur. These symptoms, common to arthritic individuals, have been effectively treated with controlled dosages of vitamin B-3.

Arthritic individuals, as well as disease-free persons, cite better sleep patterns when using niacin. Niacin is a viable alternative to using sleeping pills or tranquilizers (which promote free-radical aggression). Niacin actually binds to the same nerve cell receptors as Valium®, Libruim® or Dalmane®, popular medications to reduce anxiety. Acting as a nutrient, niacin augments this natural anxiety-reducing process instead of overriding it.

In addition, niacin today is used to treat elevated cholesterol levels. In fact, data indicates that niacin actually balances the ratio of LDL (the "bad" cholesterol) to HDL (the "good" cholesterol) in your favor. This increase in HDLs (high-density lipoproteins) in contrast to lowering LDLs (low density lipoprotein) is of great significance for the individual prone to arthritic disturbances. Evidence presented in the *New England Journal of Medicine* by Dr. Daniel Steinberg (1991) of the University of California in San Diego in a study of men throughout sixteen European cities via the World Health Organization revealed that HDL cholesterol has dynamic antioxidant capabilities. This is actually how it prevents damage to arterial walls.

As Dr. Kaufman discovered, the ability of niacin to keep arteries and blood vessels dilated was beneficial in preventing and treating arthritic disturbances as well as a number of metabolic disorders. The reason niacin is so beneficial to arthritics as dilation of the blood vessels occurs is because this facilitates the flow of oxygen and nutrients to the skin's surface. Nutrients and oxygen also are able to reach the brain and heart muscle much more efficiently. When administered daily, niacin causes a reduction in histamine production. This improves the body's ability to withstand allergic responses, and reduces natural auto-immune responses and continued destruction of valuable cartilage.

The recommended dose for niacin is based on calorie intake, 6.6 mg. per 1,000 calories. Garrison and Somer (*The Nutrition Desk Reference*, 1995) state that niacin intake should be 13 mg. daily for adults, even if food intake falls below 2,000 calories.

For continued regression and relief of symptoms, high dosages of niacin, as indicated in Dr. Kaufman's early experiments, are necessary. Current data suggests that when niacin is used in the range of 1,000 to 3,000 milligrams per day, supervision by a qualified health professional is warranted.

Contradictions

Individual suffering form diabetes, glaucoma, gout, liver disease or peptic ulcers should only use niacin under medical supervision. Also, clinical trials have shown niacin to be toxic to the liver in large dosages (over 500 to 1,000 mg.), hence the reason for close medical supervision at these ranges.

Additionally, niacin can cause a flushing sensation in some sensitive individuals. Niacinamide and inositol hexanicotinate are flush-free forms.

VITAMIN B-5

Sometimes called the "vitamin of athletes" or the "anti-stress vitamin," vitamin B-5 (calcium pantothenate) is basically an energy vitamin, and it may play a role in the energy cycle of an enzyme conversion called the Krebs Cycle or Citric Acid Cycle. As early as 1963, researchers in England found that people with rheumatoid arthritis had lower levels of B-5. Injections of B-5 were able to provide temporary relief to those arthritis sufferers.

Similar results were obtained with oral administration of vitamin B-5 by Dr. David W. Twickenham (1980, p. 211). In this study, participants were given increasing doses of B-5 until they could tolerate, without stomach upset, one 500-milligram tablet four times a day for a combined daily dose of 2,000 milligrams.

The total treatment time was eight weeks, including the first week of gradually increasing doses. The researcher reported that, "...highly significant effects were recorded for calcium pantothenate (B-5) in reducing the duration of morning stiffness, degree of disability and severity of pain." The subjects in a control group who received a placebo did not experience any such effects.

VITAMIN B-6

According to Kronhausen and associates (1989), this nutrient helps with arthritic discomfort by shrinking swollen joint membranes and dissolving rancid fat deposits. Pain is reduced and the sufferer regains some of the lost mobility in the joints. These researchers also contend that vitamin B-6 protects the insulating myelin sheath around nerves. This is another instance of B-6's ability to control pain in arthritic and rheumatoid conditions.

VITAMIN C

Vitamin C is one of the most well-known vitamins used to prevent or reduce the severity of colds. This nutrient, made famous by Linus Pauling, the chemist and Nobel Prize winner, has many biological functions besides preventing scurvy and fighting colds. Dr. Pauling, as well as the prominent researchers Cheraskin, Ringsdorf, and Sisley, maintain that most animals have the ability to manufacture their own vitamin C due to a special enzyme, I-gulonolactone oxidase. Dr. Pauling believed that through some evolutionary process we lost our ability to manufacture our own.

Since vitamin C is absolutely necessary to life and its processes, it must be supplied via the diet. For the arthritic individual, vitamin C is critical since it is responsible for the building and formation of collagen—the glue-like compound that holds bone, cartilage, ligaments, tendons and connective tissue together.

According to Dr. James Greenwood, who has served as chief of neurosurgery at Texas Methodist Hospital, large dosages of vitamin C have produced remarkable results in reducing arthritic discomfort. He attributed this to the fact that vitamin C is involved with just about all repair efforts made by the body.

Despite its remarkable properties, as a holistic health counselor I am still amazed by the number of individuals who refuse to buy vitamin C if the label contains unfamiliar words—such as "protector antioxidant." I try to educate people in how to read a label, and more importantly, to take a moment to investigate the attributes of a word or phrase that may be new on a supplement bottle.

In one of the most developed nations in the world you would assume that the health-giving attributes of antioxidants and their ability to slow down or even stop the progression of arthritis and other chronic degenerative diseases would be common knowledge. However, a 1991 Gallup Poll revealed the opposite. Only twenty-one percent of the U.S. population had any knowledge of, or had even heard the term *antioxidant*.

The Master Nutrient

Because of its diverse use and needs in the body, vitamin C is sometimes referred to as the master nutrient. According to Linus Pauling, vitamin C is different from many other nutrients. He contends that the amount that is naturally synthesized by animals is literally hundreds of times the amount people routinely obtain from foods. Pauling insists that this extra vitamin C being produced has major ramifications to maintaining optimal health, otherwise animals wouldn't be producing so much of it. For the treatment and possible prevention of arthritis alone the list of benefits is impressive. For example, vitamin C:

- Repairs and regenerates vitamin E, needed to support good circulation and capillary integrity.
- Inhibits hardening of the arteries.

- Detoxifies the liver. Healthy liver function plays a big role in our ability to decrease or minimize painful auto-immune responses.
- Acts as a strong antihistamine.
- Is essential for the strength, health, cohesion and soundness of collagen.
- Is vital to adrenal and thyroid gland function. When these two glands are compromised, this sets in motion or increases the likelihood of metabolic malfunctions, leading to increased arthritic disturbances.
- Lowers low density lipoproteins (LDLs). This will increase the antioxidant capabilities of HDLs (high density lipoproteins), thus reducing the build-up of cholesterol in arteries.
- Enhances fluid elimination and increases circulation.
- Increases wound healing and the repair of bone.
- Can increase neutrophil (white blood cell) activity, thus providing stronger immune response, and decreasing auto-immune responses.

A Natural Pain Killer

Although not thought of in terms of reducing pain, vitamin C's ability to do so is supported by scientific documentation. Vitamin C reacts to pain in a similar fashion as does aspirin, by blocking the production of the compound PGE2 and PGF2 alpha. Forget the jargon, but remember that when these prostaglandins (hormone-like substances) are activated, they cause the pain, fever, inflammation and unpleasantness that you may experience when your arthritis flares up.

Scientists now know that vitamin C calls into action a "good" prostaglandin, PGE1, to produce lymphocytes, which enhance our ability to neutralize the negative effects of the "bad" prostaglandins (PGE2 and PGF2). This is why vitamin C, in consistent daily dosages may be very beneficial, in contrast to aspirin. Aspirin focuses on pain reduction but does nothing to eliminate the cause of the pain.

Aging, Arthritis And Vitamin C

Aging increases the need for vitamin C, as does having arthritis. Unfortunately, however, about two-thirds of women of advancing age are found to be deficient, and the statistics for men are not much better. Lack of vitamin C could compromise one's ability to maintain proper nutrient levels that support immunity and encourage growth and repair of damaged cartilage.

Researchers in England, at the University of Surrey's Department of Biochemistry, studied the effects of vitamin C on the painful bone disorder known as Paget's disease. This condition occurs as a result of faulty metabolism in which bone resorption and formation processes happen at out-of-control rates. The result is bone deformity and severe pain, due to nerve fibers being crushed.

These researchers found that by taking 3000 mg. of oral ascorbic acid (vitamin C) daily for two weeks, patients had complete or partial relief of pain. Credit was given to vitamin C's essential role in the production of collagen, the natural material from which bone matrix is made. Additionally, vitamin C acts on blood vessels, reduces inflammation, and promotes the proper functioning of nerve fibers, thus reducing the sensations of pain (Basu et al., 1978).

The Right Dose

Recommended dosage of vitamin C is 60 mg. a day, set by The National Academy of Sciences. This dose is questioned by many alternative practitioners, and some conventional groups. More frequently, suggested dosages range from 500 to 3,000 mg. daily. Depending on severity of the disorder, dosages may be even higher.

In a consulting capacity to the Center for Stress, Pain and Wellness Management (Wilmington, Delaware), I generally recommend 3,000 to 5,000 mgs. of vitamin C daily, based on individual tolerance and biochemistry. I have maintained this daily range throughout the last twenty years. As a holistic healthcare instructor I generally recommend these ranges to my adult students, as well as to consumers suffering from arthritic discomfort. However, please check with a healthcare provider before starting any high dosage regimen.

Special Note: Think of vitamin C as a silent partner, working best when pain is not present, preventing disturbances before they happen. One of the biggest mistakes you could make in the use of vitamins to prevent and treat arthritic disorders is to only incorporate them during an acute episode. The most important factor in using vitamin C is its blood concentration levels. Since we are incapable of making our own steady supply, vitamin C needs to be used in equal daily dosages. It will not reduce pain as it occurs.

VITAMIN E

Vitamin E has a long history of use, and has long endured the ridicule of conventional health professionals for its use as a valuable tool in the prevention of heart disease. Current research, however, has validated this ability and has prompted more and more health officials to promote vitamin E. In fact, in a recent nationwide survey by Decision Analyst of Arlington, Texas, results revealed that one-third of all American adults routinely take vitamin E. Today, vitamin E has surpassed calcium to become the second most-used single supplement in the country, trailing only vitamin C.

Like niacin (vitamin B-3), vitamin E is a vasodilator. It promotes circulation, and has very powerful antioxidant capabilities. According to world-famous vitamin E researchers, the late Evan V. Shute, M.D. and W.E. Shute, M.D. (Wade, 1970, pp. 62-63), it produces collateral circulation around obstructed deep veins.

These researchers found that vitamin E enables tissues to better utilize oxygen, thus reducing congested debris that cause chronic leg cramps and painful phlebitic discomfort. In his clinical application of vitamin E, Dr. Evan Shute cited the following case studies of his patients:

- A forty-six-year-old woman given 600 units of vitamin E was able to resume work without pain and discomfort of her severe leg cramps. This protocol, coupled with calcium, resulted in her improvement in one month.
- An eighty-four-year-old woman suffering from protruding leg veins and arthritis throughout most of her life was administered 375 units of vitamin E a day. Within two months, she had reported that her discomfort had disappeared.

In addition to the above, research by Ayres and Mihan in 1969 revealed that patients suffering with muscular pain usually had prompt relief within ten days of consistent vitamin E usage. According to Dr. Ayres and Mihan, vitamin E helps to facilitate glycogen storage in the muscle (cited in Wade, 1970, p. 74).

As reported by H.J. Roberts, M.D. in the *Journal of the American Geriatric Society* (7:65), many patients suffering from muscular constriction, aches and pains, frequently suffer from low blood sugar. This means that individuals prone to rheumatoid arthritic dysfunction may benefit from the consistent use of vitamin E because it effectively helps to restore low glycogen levels in muscles, thus rejuvenating painful limbs, and thereby reducing the constant cycles of pain.

Furthermore, C.L. Steinberg, M.D., chief of the Arthritis Clinic of Rochester General Hospital, successfully treated over three hundred patients suffering with fibrositis (fibromyalgia) using various dose ranges of vitamin E (*Annals of the New York Academy of Science*, 10:3-69, cited by Wade).

Past and present studies have confirmed vitamin E's antioxidant abilities as well as its ability to reduce auto-immune responses. Studies have also shown vitamin E to be effective at increasing the body's ability to adapt under stress, a crucial attribute to the arthritic individual.

Vitamin E provides other attributes to arthritis sufferers. It can:

- Slow down peroxidation cycles
- Stabilize cell membrane structures
- Prevent blood clotting
- Reduce lung damage
- Slow down free-radical aggression
- Protect prostacyclin (PGI2) production (the hormone that gives our veins and arteries their Teflon®-like coating, which helps keep blood flowing).

According to Kronhausen, Kronhausen and Demopoulous (1989), vitamin E use may be warranted over aspirin and indomethacin. They point out the fact that these two drugs destroy an important enzyme in blood platelets, thus deactivating them. This is why intestinal bleeding occurs with prolonged aspirin use. Vitamin E simply prevents excessive fat oxidation that makes platelets stick together. The action of antioxidants like vitamin E prevent occlusions (closing or blocking) of blood vessels. Paradoxically, a recent study revealed that many cardiologists regularly take vitamin E, but do not encourage the same protocol for their patients.

The recommended dose for vitamin E is 30 i.u. (international units). For therapeutic action however, 200-800 i.u. is recommended.

Special Note: If you have high blood pressure or are taking anticoagulants, your dosages of vitamin E should be in the 30 to 100 i.u. range. Please consult your healthcare provider for advice.

SELENIUM

Regardless of the cause of arthritis, there is strong evidence that selenium helps relieve its symptoms. In the spring of 1980, at the Second International Symposium on Selenium in Biology and Medicine, scientists from five continents met to discuss selenium's role in the prevention of several degenerative diseases, including arthritis. Norwegian researchers reported that, "...while in rheumatoid arthritis, superoxide radicals and lipoperoxides which can be generated in the tissues and accelerate the progression of the disease, ... selenium can slow down this process" (Passwater, 1980, pp. 85-87). This positive action is thought to occur because selenium is a component of the protective enzyme glutathione peroxidase, a powerful free-radical scavenger.

ZINC

This nutrient is a biological catalyst in many enzyme systems. In a double-blind study conducted in England, Dr. Sheldon Hendler (1986) reported that a small group of patients who had not responded to conventional arthritis treatments had considerable success with zinc. Some researchers have speculated that it is possible for zinc supplements to raise the zinc level within the joints themselves, thus having an anti-inflammatory effect at the very site of the trouble.

Another physician at the Second International Symposium on Selenium in Biology and Medicine, Dr. E. Crany of Smyrna, Georgia, had already begun treating traumatic arthritis patients with selenium and the antioxidants A, C, and E, with great success.

RECOMMENDATIONS

Ongoing research affirms the health-giving benefits of antioxidants. In your quest to find the right antioxidant based on your individual needs, I strongly recommend that you first incorporate a multiple antioxidant formula as part of your program to manage your arthritic discomfort, as well as slow down its progression.

Antioxidants have the ability to repair, prevent and rejuvenate, but do not expect overnight results, as nutritional supplements are much more deliberate in their actions and may not provide immediate relief of pain. However, your goal should be long-term maintenance. Having a good, sound, antioxidant detoxification program in place could be the most important step you take in managing arthritis and related disorders.

To assess your own antioxidant status please refer to Appendix A, which contains a questionnaire to help you determine your need for additional antioxidant supplementation. Even under seemingly healthy conditions, supplementation makes good sense according to antioxidant expert, Charles A. Thomas, Ph.D., former professor of Biological Chemistry at Harvard Medical School, now Chairman of the Cell Biology Department of the Scripps Research Foundation.

In the next chapter we will review a few "accessory" supplements. While these may not be required to support life processes, new research has revealed that because of genetic imperfections, many so-called "accessory" supplements are indeed essential due to the biochemical makeup of the individual.

In many cases, "accessory" nutrients have shown to provide support in the presence of chronic degenerative conditions such as arthritis, because of the complications arthritis causes to normal metabolic processes.

4

NATURAL ACCESSORY SUPPLEMENTS

What is considered "nonessential" for most individuals may be essential for a few people who do not have adequate ability to manufacture them within their own bodies. This is called the "justification theory" that indicates, on the basis of an individual's unique genetic nature when a nonessential nutrient may become an essential nutrient.

—Jeffrey Bland, Ph.D.
Former Director, Linus Pauling Institute

For some individuals a non-essential substance can be classified as essential based on his or her specific biochemical uniqueness or need. The synopsis that follows reviews the attributes of some of these "accessory" supplements. Recent investigations have revealed that many promising arthritis-fighters are available from a variety of sources and parts of the world, and that these can provide tremendous support to the arthritic patient.

BEE PROPOLIS

Bee propolis is known as "natural penicillin" due to its ability to destroy bacteria, viruses and fungi. Propolis is the glue-like resin that bees gather from trees and plants. Many alternative and naturopathic healthcare providers today recommend propolis to enhance immune function. Much of the knowledge concerning bee propolis and its arthritis-fighting abilities comes from research carried out in Russia. Early research by Artemov (1959) revealed that bee venom, when injected into arthritic joints, stimulated pituitary and adrenal gland action. This resulted in a natural increase of "cortisone" output. Synthetic cortisone injected into arthritic joints is a popular conventional arthritic treatment today.

The ability of bee propolis to lessen the severity of arthritic disturbances is due to its high flavonoid content. Propolis also contains high concentrations of pantothenic acid and niacin. As we previously noted in Chapter 3, both niacin and pantothenic acid can reduce the pain and discomfort associated with arthritis.

Special Note: Some individuals are prone to allergic reactions from bee pollens or bee stings. Sensitivity of this nature should be considered before using bee propolis or any bee pollen products.

BOVINE TRACHEAL CARTILAGE

Bovine trachea is the windpipe of a young cow. It is a cartilaginous part containing substances called glucosaminoglycans. Humans have these substances too. These body nutrients are sometimes considered the "glue of life" because they are part of a group of complex carbohydrates functioning mainly as structural components in connective tissue. Bovine tracheal cartilage provides two useful forms of glycosaminoglycans: chondroitin-4-sulfates and chondroitin-6-sulfates (formally called Sulfate A and C). Chondroitin sulfate enhances repair of osteoarthritis cartilage by inhibiting the enzymes that degrade cartilage.

BROMELIN

Bromelin comes from uncooked pineapple. Dallas Cloutatre, Ph.D., a well-known researcher, author and former professor of nutrition at the University of California, Berkeley, states that "…bromelin has shown the ability to improve the body's response to inflammation and swelling. This is due, in part, to its ability to possibly block the production of prostaglandins, the hormones responsible for much of the inflammation you may be experiencing" (Cloutatre, 1997, pp. 35-36).

CAYENNE PEPPER

Many arthritics, including myself, claim that cayenne (capsicum frute scens) stimulates circulation and reduces inflammation and stiffness in joints. Scientific studies have validated these claims. Steven Foster (1996, pp. 20-21) reported that topical creams of capsicum applied to affected joints effectively reduced pain. Also, a recent study conducted at the famous Mayo Clinic revealed capsicum's ability to combat pain. This is due to capsicum's ability to lower the levels of a compound called "substance P" which signals pain messages to the brain.

CHAMOMILE

This herb has a long history and is commonly used to calm the nerves, soothe the system and aid in digestion. In Europe, chamomile is consumed in tea form at a rate of a million cups a day. Many Americans use it to induce restful sleep or to reduce stress. Recent research has shown that chamomile possesses powerful compounds that reduce the activity of prostaglandins—the agents that cause much of the inflammation experienced in weakened joints. Chamomile can be purchased as a tea, in capsules, or in tincture (liquid) form.

CoQ10

This is a vitamin-like nutrient that functions as a coenzyme and triggers thousands of essential biochemical reactions. Most biochemists know CoQ10 as "ubiquinone." According to Karl

Folkers, Ph.D., winner of the Priestly Medal (the American Chemical Society's highest award), if people ask their doctors about CoQ10, they will probably say that they have never heard of it.

CoQ10's key role is in producing adenosine triphosphate (ATP), needed for energy production in every cell of the body. Secondary to that, CoQ10 functions as a powerful antioxidant.

Although CoQ10 occurs widely in our food supply, it is not always in significant amounts. In addition, each cell in the body manufactures it, though not always efficiently. According to Folkers, therapeutic dosages of CoQ10 for serious diseases range from 200 mg. to 400 mg. daily, ideally under a physician's supervision. It works in diverse conditions because the basic underlying mechanisms are the same—energy production at the cellular level and antioxidant protection against free radicals. Case studies demonstrating the dramatic effect of CoQ10 can be found in *Biophysical Research Communications* (Jan 15, 1993, 182: 247-531), and the *Clinical Investigator*, (Aug 1993, 715:134-6).

CURCUMINOIDS

Curcuminoids are a group of compounds found in the herb turmeric. Because of its bright yellow color, turmeric is used to color foods. Recent research has revealed that this substance has potent antioxidant properties, can detoxify the blood, reduce elevated cholesterol levels, kill parasites and promote bile flow from the liver.

The anti-inflammatory capabilities of curcuminoids are attributed to a group of curcuminoids that work in unison, known as the C-3 complex. This complex has demonstrated results comparable in action to several NSAID (non-steroidal anti-inflammatory) drugs. Curcuminoids work by stopping the release of inflammatory compounds originating from arachidonic acid—a fatty acid that is found primarily in animal products that increase leukotriene production. As we have learned, leukotrienes play a major role in activating allergic and inflammatory responses. It is here that curcuminoids would be of great benefit because of their ability to elevate the body's own natural anti-inflammatory actions.

For chronic conditions, 1,000 milligrams a day is recommended, or up to an ounce (4 tablespoons) of powder.

Special Note: Because of the possible problems associated with arachidonic acid production, alternative practitioners strongly recommend the elimination of animal products from the diet.

DL-PHENYLALANINE

Known as DLPA for short, this nutrient works by intensifying and prolonging your body's own natural pain-killing mechanisms. When pain occurs, brain hormones called endorphins are produced. Endorphins have similar properties to morphine, a powerful analgesic drug. Certain enzymes in the body tend to neutralize the endorphins, but DLPA inhibits the action of those enzymes, allowing endorphins a longer lifespan in which to counter pain naturally.

Hatfield and Zucker (1990) recommend taking 750 milligrams three times daily, fifteen to thirty minutes before meals. These researchers maintain that at this dose range pain begins to subside anywhere from four days to two to three weeks. The degree and level of pain reduction, ranging from mild to a general lessening of pain, may vary from individual to individual.

According to Hatfield and Zucker, less than fifteen percent of users experience no relief. In this case, these researchers suggest doubling the initial dosage for another two or three weeks. The prominent biochemical researchers Pearson and Shaw (1982, p. 186) remind us, however, that in some individuals DL-phenylalanine can increase blood pressure. They recommend starting out with a lower dosage (100mg.), especially for individuals who have high blood pressure, with daily monitoring of blood pressure levels. Dosage can then be adjusted based on individual tolerance and safety.

As cited by Pearson and Shaw, under normal circumstances, there are no toxic side effects with this supplement's use. It is advisable, however, to check with your healthcare professional when using the large dosages cited by Hatfield and Zucker.

ENZYMES

While enzymes have been used to treat a number of digestive disorders, they have gained notoriety as a valuable alternative in fighting arthritis. Enzymes are found in every inch of the body and act as catalysts. Without enzymes, the human body is essentially a pile of worthless chemicals. Enzymes keep metabolic activity alive everywhere in the body, including the joints. Without the work they do, we would die. Unfortunately, aging inhibits enzyme production and diminishes their therapeutic ability. A sixty-year-old person could have fifty percent fewer enzymes that a thirty-year-old. Fewer enzymes not only mean a possible increase in arthritic disturbances, but a host of other metabolic disorders.

Dr. Edward Howell, an early pioneer of enzyme therapy, cited a seven-year study of 700 patients suffering from rheumatoid arthritis, osteoarthritis and fibrositis (now called fibromyalgia). The patients were given seven capsules daily of a dried enzyme extract, taken after meals. In a series of 556 cases of varying types of arthritis, 283 were much improved, 219 were improved to a less extent. Of 292 cases of rheumatoid arthritis, 264 showed improvement in varying degrees.

Enzymes are probably one of the most effective, and safe alternatives you could incorporate as part of your daily supplement routine. In fact, Dr. Michael Williams, Professor of Medicine at Northwestern University and Dr. David Lopez, an associate clinical Professor of Medicine at the University of California, maintain that enzymes have an immense potential for maintaining health.

Because our supply of these powerful agents can decline with age, researchers (such as Dr. Williams and Dr. Lopez as well as Doctors Michael Murray and Joseph Pizzorno of Bastyr College), recommend the use of enzymes, especially after age forty.

EVENING PRIMROSE OIL

The evening primrose originated in North America and botanists first brought the plant from Virginia to Europe in 1614. In 1919, the *Archives of Pharmacology* published a report by Heiduschka and Luft, who were the first to do a detailed analysis of the oil extracted from the primrose plant. Current research shows that the oil of the evening primrose converts in the body to a physiologically active substance called prostaglandin E1 (PEG1). The unique quality of evening primrose oil is that it contains a substance called gamma linolenic acid (GLA), which eventually converts in the body to PEG1. In rheumatoid arthritis, the body is producing too little of these PEG1s.

Several studies on animals suggest that evening primrose oil may be helpful in human rheumatoid arthritis. Dr. Robert Zurier and his group of researchers from the University of Pennsylvania School of Medicine are credited with pioneering the belief that prostaglandin E1 acts as an anti-inflammatory (Graham, 1984). PEG1 can inhibit experimental (adjuvant) arthritis in rats, control the systematic lupus-like syndrome in mice, activate T-lymphocytes and control lysosomal enzyme release in humans. Currently, there are over one hundred clinical trials in progress. Several companies around the world market evening primrose oil products.

GARLIC

Animal studies demonstrate that garlic exhibits anti-inflammatory activity, which accounts for its effectiveness in the treatment of arthritis. In a study with rats, allisotin, prepared from garlic (200

72

mg/100g/day), was found effective against an inflammatory arthritis condition induced by formalin (formaldehyde) (Airola, 1978, pp. 18-19). Also, free-radical formation and resulting cell damage, found in arthritis and other degenerative diseases, have been neutralized by A.G.E. (Aged Garlic Extracts). Dr. Robert Lin and associates used tbutylhydroperoxide (a free-radical generator) to oxidize red blood cells, resulting in darkening of the hemoglobin and rupturing of the cells. Researchers found that adding A.G.E. to the red blood cell suspension (prior to oxidant exposure) minimized oxidation and cell rupture (*Abstracts of the First World Congress on the Health Significance of Garlic and Garlic Constituents*, 1990, p. 22).

Additionally, Professor Lau of Loma Linda University (1989) found that aged garlic extract protected lymphocytes from irradiation damage. Fresh garlic, however, had no protective effect. Furthermore, the safety of A.G.E. has been confirmed by a wide variety of toxicological tests, as well as clinical studies conducted on more than 1,000 subjects.

GINKGO BILOBA

The ginkgo biloba is one of the oldest living trees, dating back more than 200 million years. It has survived the ice age, the atomic bombing of Hiroshima, and seems to be immune to the common ravishes of nature. As one of the most widely researched compounds, ginkgo biloba today is used to treat a wide variety of ailments that are related to advancing age and degenerative decline. In fact, as one of Europe's most widely-prescribed substances, ginkgo sales total over $500 million a year. Some of the disorders that ginkgo is used to treat and possibly prevent are:

- Heart muscle injury
- Macular degeneration (blindness)
- Free-radical proliferation

- Circulatory disorders
- Ringing in the ears
- Asthma attacks

- Lipid (fat) peroxidation of cell membranes
- Platelet aggregation (possibly preventing heart attacks).

Many of ginkgo's positive attributes are thought to occur because of their ability to promote circulation throughout the system. For the arthritic, the promotion of peripheral circulation can provide increased energy and new vim and vigor to affected joints. Ginkgo's antioxidant capabilities, and its use as a viable alternative in the treatment of arthritic disturbances is attributed to its flavonoid content.

One of the researchers studying the effects of poor thyroid function is Raphael Kellerman, M. D., a New York City physician who specializes in thyroid-related conditions. According to Dr. Kellerman there are over fifty health problems related to the improper functioning of the thyroid gland. In reference to arthritic disturbances, rheumatic pain, weight gain, muscle aches and weakness, anemia and constipation, are all related to poor thyroid function (Leviton, 1998).

Additionally, ginkgo is as effective as conventional drugs in relieving the pain associated with intermittent claudication—a very painful leg condition that results when cholesterol deposits cause the arteries to narrow.

Special Note: When purchasing ginkgo biloba, please make sure the label states that it is standardized to have twenty-four percent ginkgo flavoneglycosides. This assures that the active compound in ginkgo is indeed present.

KOMBUCHA

Kombucha is a widely used tea-based beverage, fermented with the use of a "mushroom" that is actually part of a variety of different elements from yeast and bacteria (Balch and Balch, 1993, p. 56). The beverage is used to treat gastrointestinal disorders. Recent research has revealed that kombucha has powerful anti-arthritic properties. According to Dr. Morton Walker (1996), a well-known medical journalist, the reason kombucha is so effective as an alternative treatment against chronic joint inflammation is its glucuronic acid content. As cited by Dr. Walker, glucuronic acid is a precursor to the formation of glycosaminoglycan—the components in tissues that bind with water and ensure good function of connective tissue and proper joint lubrication.

Researchers maintain that once toxins and debris in weakened or functional joints attach to glucuronic acid, they are unable to be reabsorbed back into the tissues.

MANGANESE

Manganese is a trace mineral that plays a role in activating numerous enzymes. It acts as a catalyst in the synthesis of fatty acids and is necessary for normal skeletal development. Low manganese levels may cause atherosclerosis. Manganese deficiency has been implicated in tardive dyskinesia, a neuromuscular disease. Dr. George C. Cotzia, who developed the use of levo-dopa in Parkinsonism, reported at the First Annual Conference on Trace Substances in Environmental Health (1967) at the University of Missouri that manganese was necessary for the enzymatic syntheses of a material called mucopolysaccharide, which is deficient in rheumatoid arthritis.

Mucopolysaccharides are lubricating substances naturally present in cartilage. The National Research Council sets adequate dietary intake at 2.5 to 5 milligrams a day for adults.

METHYL-SULFONYL-METHANE

This sulfur-based compound, M.S.M., has received much attention in recent years. A normal by-product of dimethyl sulfoxide, commonly known as DSMO, M.S.M. has powerful pain-killing and anti-inflammatory properties. Providing much of the body's sulfur needs is what gives it its dynamic properties. Sulfur is responsible for building what scientists call disulfide bonds. When these are formed they help hold tissue together and assist in the preservation and formation of protein, collagen and glucosamine (the building blocks of cartilage).

The pain-reducing effects of M.S.M. were recently confirmed in a trial of sixteen patients in a double-blind study. After being administered 2250 mg. of M.S.M. per day, eighty percent of the participants were better able to control their pain. Additionally, as cited by Jack Challem (1998), known as "the nutrition reporter," in one of three different case studies, a priest from Frenchville, Pennsylvania, who suffered from bursitis, as well as arthritic problems in his knees, was able to resume normal activity after about a year of M.S.M. The priest commented that his usual pain and discomfort returned when he stopped his daily regimen of M.S.M.

MILK THISTLE

This herb is used extensively to cleanse and detoxify the liver. Silymarin, as it is also referred to, can be categorized as a flavonoid with potent antioxidant capabilities. Milk thistle has the ability to slow down the formation of free radicals and those destructive inflammatory compounds called leukotrienes.

OMEGA-3 FISH OIL

The present popularity of fish oils dates back to a study by two Danish scientists, John Dyerberg and Hans Olaf Bang (1978). They compared the effects of the typical, high-saturated-fat, high-cholesterol diet of the Danes with the high-marine-oil diet of the Greenland Eskimos. Omega-3 fish oils consist of eicosapentanoic (EPA) and docosahexanoic acid (DHA) which are the beneficial factors of these special types of fats, with strong anti-inflammatory properties. Dyerberg and Bang found that the Eskimos not only had less coronary heart disease than Americans, Europeans and even contemporary Japanese, they also suffered less from chronic inflammatory disorders such as rheumatoid arthritis, which is practically unknown to them. Data revealed that this was due to their higher intake of marine oils—the omega-3 fatty acids EPA and DHA.

Dr. Joel M. Kremer and colleagues (1987) in the division of rheumatology at Albany Medical College in New York have been able to duplicate this anti-inflammatory effect by supplementing the diets of rheumatoid arthritis patients with 1.8 grams of EPAs and DHAs provided by MAX-EPA capsules daily for fourteen weeks. The result was that the fish oils produced, as researchers put it, "subjective alleviation of active rheumatoid arthritis." Also, researchers at Harvard University found that 1.8 grams of EPA greatly improved tenderness in the joints, and morning stiffness in individuals suffering from rheumatoid arthritis (cited in Quillin, 1987). Improvements in this study group occurred most noticeably within twelve weeks.

The results of this study can be attributed to the fact that when EPA and DHA are high in the diet, there is a corresponding reduction in leukotriene production. As previously noted, leukotrienes cause inflammation in the tissues.

SEA CUCUMBER

A new product currently under investigation is a defensive toxin discharged by the marine animal known as the sea cucumber. When these toxins are taken orally, they have been found to be effective anti-inflammatory agents. Recently, Australia's Department of Health approved sea cucumber as an effective arthritis treatment. A study done at the University of Queensland Medical Center by Ron A. Hazelton, M.D. found that sea cucumber was also anti-arthritic, helping to reverse the disease process rather than just curtail the symptoms.

SHARK CARTILAGE

Shark carilage is one of the most talked about new products in the health market. Dr. William Lane, author of *Sharks Don't Get Cancer* (1992) reported the miraculous effects of the active substance in shark cartilage on the popular TV program, *60 Minutes*. As early as 1971, glucosamine sulfate, an amino monosaccharide naturally present in cartilage, had shown the ability to restore the proper chemistry and rebuild or heal osteoarthritic cartilage (*Pharmacology*, 1971, 5:337). Shark cartilage actually inhibits the formation of new blood vessels.

As we have discussed previously, angiogenesis plays a major role in causing many degenerative joint conditions. According to Dr. Lane, once shark cartilage is in a person's bloodstream, its anti-inflammatory and anti-angiogenic characteristics begin to work. Angiogenesis has also been implicated in the stoppage of tumor growth by destroying the network of blood vessels that tumors need for nourishment and to remove waste products. Recently, Dr. Lane received full FDA permission to do phase II clinical trials on humans for advanced non-responsive prostate cancer.

WHITE WILLOW BARK

This herb is the original source of aspirin's active ingredient, salicylic acid. Over centuries this substance has been used against many painful conditions including headaches, rheumatism, neuralgia, arthritis, gout and angina. White willow can be purchased over the counter, and is usually sold in capsule form. Please follow manufacturer's guidelines on dosage.

YUCCA

This desert plant is a genus of trees belonging to the liliaceae family, and Native Americans used yucca for many purposes. John W. Yale, Ph.D., a botanical biochemist, extracted the steroid saponin, and collaborated in clinical trials of its efficacy with the

National Arthritis Medical Clinic in Desert Hot Springs, California (1973). A one-year study was conducted. Of the 165 participants tested, forty-nine percent reported favorably, twenty-eight percent felt no change or effect, and twenty-three percent could not decide. More than sixty percent stated that they experienced less pain, stiffness and swelling, the three major complaints of arthritis, and thirty-nine percent reported that they felt no change. The effects were felt in four days to three months. Dosage varied, averaging four tablets daily, taken before, during and after meals (Mindell, 1978, p. 51).

OTHER AGENTS

Yoshihide Hagiwana, M.D. ("Green Waves of Barley Ease Arthritis For Some," 1995) has revealed potent anti-inflammatory activity of barley-juice components.

Recent extensive scientific research studies showed that the herb boswellia (taken internally or used externally in a cream) is extremely beneficial for arthritis and rheumatic diseases. Ayurvedic (the medical system of India) medical texts for the last 1,500 years have strongly praised the anti-inflammatory, anti-arthritic and anti-pain qualities of boswellia serrata (see: Safyh, 1996, and Singh, 1986).

Additionally, scientists are conducting research on alfalfa, and herbs such as devil's claw, angelica root, cinnamon twig and licorice.

NATURAL BORN ARCHITECTS

When nonsteroidal anti-inflammatory drugs are used (aspirin, ibuprofen, Motrin®), these medications can actually stop cartilage formation. Current data has substantiated that these drugs also speed the destruction of this valuable cartilage. Researchers have recently found that when certain naturally-occurring substances were orally administered they actually helped to stimulate the production of new connective tissue. Three such products are: chondroitin sulfate, glucosamine sulfate, and cetyl myristoleate (CMO). These products do not require a doctor's prescription. They can be purchased in health food and drug stores across the U.S. A brief synopsis of each follows.

Chondroitin Sulfate

Chondroitins are naturally-occurring substances that interfere with the production of certain enzymes that can break down cartilage. Chondroitins also help attract fluid, thus keeping joints lubricated. According to Jason Theodosakis, M.D., author of *The Arthritis Cure* (1997), besides drawing fluid to arthritic joints, chondroitin:

1. Protects existing cartilage from premature breakdown
2. Interferes with other enzymes that inhibit proper nutrient transport to cartilage
3. Stimulates the production of proteoglycans (large, water-binding molecules), chondroitins and glycomasaminoglycans known as GAG's (proteins in cartilage that bind the water in the cartilage), which are molecules that serve as building blocks for healthy new cartilage.

Based on his experience and study of chondroitin sulfates, Dr. Theodosakis has found dosages of 1.5 to 10 grams per day to be safe. Also, there is an added plus in this equation, chondroitin works very well with glycocyamine sulfate.

Glucosamine Sulfate

Glucosamine sulfate is the key material that determines how may proteoglycan molecules are produced in the cartilage. When adequate glucosamine is present, proteoglycan production increases. Glucosamine's main function is to hasten the manufacture of connective tissue. Think of this connective tissue as a super fiber optic network that holds your joints together. Being the primary substance of that network, glucosamine production is critical to good joint health.

As we age, our ability to produce and maintain adequate levels of glycocyamine sulfate diminishes. When levels begin to drop, cartilage loses its ability to hold water, thus causing much friction between joints. This occurrence can be compared to blowing out the shock absorbers on your car. As cited by Julian Whitaker, M.D., a well-known medical professional who incorporates sound alternative therapies into his practice, 1.5 grams of glucosamine in head-to-head trials against 1.2 grams of ibuprofen (the active ingredient in Motrin®, Advil®, and Nuprin®) have revealed some astonishing results. Researchers at the Saint John's Hospital in Oporto, Portugal found that within the first two weeks of use, glucosamine had a definite advantage in reducing pain. However, after eight weeks the subjects who used the ibuprofen showed increased signs of reoccurring pain and discomfort, while the glucosamine group showed a regression of pain and symptoms. In fact, this gradual regression started to appear within four weeks (Whitaker, 1995, pp. 311-314). While glucosamine took longer for initial results to occur, its actions preserved and nurtured an environment for long-term use and effectiveness.

Ray Sahelian, M.D., an internationally known expert in the field of natural hormone therapy and the use of natural supplements in treating chronic degenerative ailments, states that patients usually see results from glucosamine within four months. He suggests dose ranges of 500 mg. to 1,000 mg. three times a day for a few months, followed by a daily dose of 500 mg. for maintenance.

Cetyl Myristoleate

Cetyl myristoleate is found in vegetables and legumes, and was first discovered and isolated at the National Institutes of Health in

1971. Cetyl myristoleate (CMO) has gained national attention. In human trials, this substance has shown a remarkable ability to:

- Act as sort of a super lubricant for joints, muscles and other tissues throughout the body
- Function as an immune system modulator, by stimulating certain immunoglobulin, which are part of the body's natural defense system.

Researchers believe that the above feature has enormous potential in diminishing or controlling the auto-immune response of arthritic discomfort and controlling prostaglandin activity. Prostaglandins are hormones responsible for childbirth and labor, menstruation, blood clotting and the stimulation of the immune system. Prostaglandins also are intimately involved with the inflammatory response that can cause much pain and distress.

As cited by Ken Babal (1997), a certified nutritionist, in a 1996 multi-center one month clinical study with 431 diagnosed arthritic patients with various forms of arthritis, CMO showed some remarkable results. When combined with glucosamine hydrochloride, sea cucumber, and hydrolyzed cartilage, an eighty-three percent improvement was shown in test subjects (Kremer, 1996). Babal observed that if a new prescription drug produced these kinds of results, or was even fifty percent effective, it would make headlines in a matter of days.

Special Note: The problem here is that drug companies are unable to patent naturally-occurring substances. When a drug company gets exclusive rights to market a medicine, it has a monopoly on it, they and they alone have the exclusive rights to manufacture and distribute it for seventeen years. Hence their reluctance to pursue the attributes of alternative, naturally-occurring substances.

An Anecdotal Success Story

As a sixty-two-year-old office worker, Mark had failing arthritic knees, and was slated to have both knees replaced. He wanted to wait until retirement to have the procedure done, but the pain was becoming unbearable. Mark loved tennis, yet because of his pain he was losing his will to play. After a few rounds on the court, and in the aftermath, severe swelling and pain left him incapacitated for days.

After reviewing the possible merits of chondroitin and glucosamine sulfate, Mark decided to try these supplements for six months before proceeding with the surgery. In addition to the above products, I suggested to Mark that he also try a new proprietary product called the CM System™, namely cetyl myristoleate. Additional products found within this system are hydrolyzed gelatin, sea cucumber and glucosamine sulfate.

In using the CM System™ it is recommended that individuals initially go through what is known as a "loading phase." This phase consists of a thirty-day period of taking one capsule in the CM System™ before each meal. After this cycle was over, Mark stayed on a daily maintenance dose of 500 mg. of glycosamine sulfate and chondroitin sulfate, and began to see some slight improvements in less than six months. His range of mobility had improved and his morning stiffness was less severe. The most noticeable change was his ability to return to the tennis court. He still had pain, but not the excruciating or debilitating type as before, and without the severe swelling. Although Mark knew that he would never cure his arthritis, he did wonder what his quality of life may have been like if he had started this regimen some years ago.

The CM System™ is available in major vitamin and health food stores, and can be purchased without a doctor's prescription.

IN SUPPORT OF SUPPLEMENTS

Ray Sahelian, M.D. (1997, p. 6) asks a probing question:

When I reviewed the clinical studies done on glucosamine over the years, I noticed something very unusual. There were no studies done in the U.S.! All of them were done by researchers in Italy, the Philippines, Thailand, Germany, Portugal and other foreign countries. Why is this?

According to Dr. Sahelian, U.S. pharmaceutical companies are not going to spend millions of dollars researching natural supplements that they will never have the exclusive rights to.

Mary Ann Block, D.O., author of *No More Ritalin: Treating Attention Deficient Hyperactivy Disorder Without Drugs*, states that, in her experience, "many times dietitians, like physicians, will often reflect their own educational bias when they tell us we don't need supplements" (1996, p. 111).

Dr. Andrew Weil (1995, p. 50-51), one of the country's most well-known and well-respected physicians, and an expert in alternative medicine, makes the following statement:

Talking about herbal cures with doctors is particularly difficult because they have no training in medical botany. Take ginkgo biloba for example. Dozens of scientific articles based on both animal and human experiments have appeared in good, peer review journals, although the journals are not ones read by American physicians. I cannot think of one physician who reads *Plant Medica*, a German journal and one of the best.

At the New York Academy of Sciences' 1992 symposium, "Beyond Deficiency: New Views on the Function and Health Effects of Vitamins," Lawrence Machlin, Ph.D., Director of

Human Research, Hoffman-LaRoche stated in his introductory remarks:

> Historically, nutritionists have been concerned with vitamins in terms of their role in preventing vitamin deficiency diseases, and their bio-chemical role as coenzymes. Research is rapidly accumulating that this is a very limited view and that vitamins have significant health effects beyond preventing deficiency diseases...These findings have made it necessary to reexamine the criteria used to establish recommended levels of vitamin consumption and to determine what is meant by optimal intake. (669: 1-92)

ASSESSING YOUR OWN SUPPLEMENT STATUS

When you review the remarks make by Lawrence Machlin, Ph.D. and the other prominent health professionals it is clear that current thinking and data encourages the use of supplements. Many natural supplements covered in this chapter and throughout this book are viable alternatives to the NSAID drugs that not only have serious side effects but also promote free-radical aggression and actually speed up the destructive processes that degrade tissues and joints.

To assess your own nutrient status, there are two inexpensive tests that you may consider; each of which may be covered by some health insurance including Medicare.

1. *Pantox Antioxidant Profile*™: This test measures twenty different nutritional factors that determine the effectiveness of the body's antioxidant system. This test will help you determine if you are getting the right antioxidants in the correct

ratios. For more information on this test contact: Pantox Laboratories, 4622 Santa Fe Street, San Diego, CA 92109; 1-888-726-8698 or 1-619-272-3885.

2. *Functional Intracellular Analysis*™: This test looks at levels of vitamins, minerals, antioxidants, amino acids and fatty acids. It actually measures how well these nutrients are functioning within live white blood cells, versus what is considered to be an acceptable level of those nutrients in those cells. If the cells are not utilizing or metabolizing nutrients properly, appropriate cell functions can be compromised (*Alternative Medicine Digest*, "Energizing Chronic Fatigue," #19, Sept. 1997, 63).

For the arthritic individual, poor nutrient selection as well as improper utilization of nutrients can stimulate unwanted inflammatory responses. This compromise of nutrients can possibly cause the proliferation of free-radical aggression, thus perpetuating the on and off cycle of chronic pain.

To find out more about this test contact Spectra Cell Laboratories, Inc., 515 Post Oak Blvd., Suite 830, Houston, TX 77027; 1-713-621-3101 or 1-800-227-5227.

In addition to the above, a new kit known as the *Vitamed*™ test can be used to test your nutritional status at home (*Alternative Medicine Digest*, "Natural Pharmacy," Issue #25, July 1998, 65-66).

With the *Vitamed*™ test you send in urine samples and within ten days you get a detailed analysis of specific levels of nutrients. Three tests, which can be done separately or as a complete analysis, detail vitamin and mineral levels as well as your ability to handle free radicals. For more information contact: Medical Direct Corporation, 22722 Vistawood Way, Boca Raton, FL, 33428; 1-800-658-2227 or 1-516-483-0375.

YOU ARE YOUR BEST TEACHER

Biomedical researchers Pearson and Shaw assert that finding the right antioxidant or combination of supplements that works for you will happen only through trial and error. The famed orthomolecular nutritional scientists Hoffer and Walker express a similar viewpoint. They relate that the medical use of supplements has essentially focused on prevention and treatment of deficiencies, whereas the use of much larger amounts to treat conditions not related to deficiencies has been much less. Furthermore, such treatment hasn't been tested on a large scale.

Hoffer and Walker also maintain that the efficacy of the right individual regimen has to occur only one way—by trial and error, through self experimentation.

Before incorporating any new supplement regimen I strongly advise you to consult with your healthcare professional, especially if you are already taking any prescription drugs. It is important to remember that in the world of supplements, excessive dosages are not always better. In many cases, the combination of many different nutrients and accessory compounds working together is more beneficial than one large dose of a single substance. The beauty of natural supplementation is the positive synergistic effect that multiple supplements can have.

In a recent discussion with a woman who suffered from rheumatoid arthritis, she revealed that she had opted to "tough it out" without the conventional medication prescribed because of unpleasant side effects. She admitted that her attacks were more frequent in the summer months than in the winter months. This confused her because many of her friends who also had rheumatoid arthritis complained that their symptoms were much more severe in the winter or colder months. I asked her if there was something she was eating differently in the summer than in the winter, and asked her to start a daily diary, explaining that one of the best things she could do for herself was to become a "food cop." I recommended that she start recording what foods she was eating and her reactions to them, as well as to become more cognizant of her activities and any subsequent flare-ups. When you the individual know what clues to look for, the signals that precipitate the pain and discomfort of your symptoms can be alleviated by you!

In the next chapter, "Food Is Your Best Medicine," we will take a look at how food can help, or in many cases hinder, your efforts to gain control and better manage your particular arthritic problem. Understanding how and what foods could be at the root of your problem should be a primary concern to anyone suffering from arthritic disturbances.

5

FOOD IS YOUR BEST MEDICINE

Arthritis is made worse by our own incorrect eating habits. It has been amply demonstrated that our health destroying foods are largely the cause of a whole class of degenerative diseases. What arthritis and all these diseases have in common is that they are not caused by a virus or bacterium that can be destroyed by drugs. They are often activated by our life-wrecking eating habits.

—Lauri M. Aesoph, N.D.

Growing numbers of researchers and health experts advocate that a diet rich in vegetables (cooked and raw) can play a major role in the ability to combat, and in some cases regress, the debilitating effects of arthritis. Fruits such as bananas, sour cherries and pineapples have also been shown to reduce pain and inflammation. Besides knowing what to eat, learning which foods we are sensitive to can go a long way in alleviating, but more importantly preventing, the onset of an attack of arthritis.

Many researchers advise arthritis sufferers to avoid meat, fish, cow's milk, cheese and sugar. The late Carlton Fredericks insisted that the family of nightshade foods—tomatoes, peppers (all types except black), potatoes, and eggplant—should be eliminated from the diet. In addition, studies have shown that when processed foods are eliminated from the diet, many arthritic individuals remain free of symptoms. Neal Barnard, M.D., President of the Physicians' Committee for Responsible Medicine in Washington D.C. and his associates have duplicated these findings. According to Dr. Barnard "...it is not exactly known why, but when animal food sources are eliminated from patient diet regimens, in many cases their arthritis will go into complete remission," (1998, pp. 80-86). He went on to say that the elimination of dairy products can be of great benefit in winning against the effects of this debilitating disease.

DIGESTING PROTEIN—A PROBLEM FOR MANY

Most cooked foods enter the stomach at a temperature of more than 104 degrees, and this heat can destroy some of the gastric enzymes needed for digestion. Liquids consumed at the same time can delay protein digestion by further reducing the concentration of gastric juices.

Many people, especially arthritics, cannot digest meat properly because of a deficiency in the pancreatic enzymes, bile and hydrochloric acid. As a point of reference, pancreatin is a term used to describe enzymes secreted to digest a certain type of foods. During the digestive process, pancreatic enzyme secretions of lipase, protease and amylase occur. Lipase enzymes digest fats, protease digest proteins and amylase digest carbohydrates.

Bile acids, which emanate from the liver, work to emulsify (i.e., break down) fat, while hydrochloric acid dissolves food particles and kills many harmful microorganisms. When HCL (hydrochloric acid) is secreted into the stomach, it aids in protein digestion.

The problem with animal protein is that the excess amounts not used for growth and repair are not utilized properly. This unused portion can cause the accumulation of uric acid, a waste by-product of protein metabolism. When this waste product begins to accumulate faster than normal excretory cycles can handle, it can lodge in joints causing severe pain and discomfort. In fact, studies have shown that the excess uric acid left in the body from any one meal could lead to an acute attack of gout, rheumatism or arthritis. This is due in part to the fact that the human liver and kidneys combined have a limited capacity to get rid of only about eight grains of uric acid in a twenty-four hour period. Consuming as little as a pound of highly concentrated animal protein from meat and meat by-products (hotdogs, lunch meats, etc.), can generate as much as eighteen grains of uric acid. (One ounce equals 437.5 grains.)

Researchers today know that milk and milk by-products are among the foods that most commonly trigger the pain and discomfort of arthritis. Mucus, which accumulates from processed, baked and pasteurized dairy products, can deposit in tissues, clog blood vessels, cause deterioration of blood vessel walls, and thereby cause blood velocity to slow down. When this happens, needed nutrients may not reach proper organs, with undigested particles finding a home in weakened areas, namely the joints. The mucus build-up that can occur in the digestive tract is made worse by milk.

The accumulation of mucus can also contribute to over acidity of the body, and activate acute arthritic disturbances. Furthermore, prolonged action can cause dissolution of bone calcium. This calcium, plus ingested inorganic minerals, are carried by the bloodstream looking for a drop-off point—inevitably in the joints. Most people fail to realize that arthritis can kill, according to Robert Wilner, M.D., of the Pain Center in North Miami Beach, Florida. In severe cases, arthritis may affect not only bones and joints, but also blood vessels, kidneys, skin, eyes and the brain.

If you must drink milk, many herbalists recommend adding papaya tablets to the milk. The papaya will help reduce mucus buildup, and the cow's milk will then more closely resemble the constitutionality of breast milk, in turn, increasing its digestibility.

THE LEAKY-GUT CONNECTION

In scientific terms, the "Leaky-Gut" is known as the Malabsorption Syndrome. This occurs when food particles that wouldn't normally cross the intestinal lining enter the body, creating unwanted immune responses. Recognizing these particles as foreign objects, the body begins to attack its own tissues. This insidious phenomenon (as we noted in Chapter 1) is known as an auto-immune response. In leaky gut situations the permeability of the intestines is severely compromised—a situation comparable to driving on a sunny day with your convertible top down, only to be drenched in a rainstorm when the top fails to go up. This internal malady can be tremendously problematic to those suffering from arthritic complications.

This malabsorption syndrome, in the absence of arthritic disturbances, could also be considered as a long-term causative factor associated with the step-by-step progression to initial onset of arthritis. Furthermore, there is evidence that conventional medicines used to treat osteoarthritis and rheumatoid arthritis accelerate the negative aspects of the leaky gut syndrome.

INCREASING CALCIUM SOLUBILITY

Although arthritics have been told to stay away from sodium (salt), this element has some very important responsibilities. Organic sodium has the ability to increase the solubility of calcium, making it usable for its intended function—i.e., to build strong bones and to support many different metabolic processes. Also, when organic sodium is present, it helps maintain an alkaline internal environment versus the destructive nature of an acid one.

Your alkaline reserve is made up of minerals that neutralize the negative effects of acid-producing foods, such as animal protein and dairy products. These foods have been implicated in increasing the onset and severity of various arthritic disturbances.

The more protein and dairy products you consume, the more energy your body must produce to prepare for waste elimination. The end product of this attempt to reduce the waste by-products is "acid ash."

Some of the best sources of increasing the body's pool of organic sodium are fruits and vegetables, not sodium chloride (common table salt).

THE ACID-ALKALINE BALANCE

Many people wonder what being alkaline instead of acidic has to do with arthritis, and why is it important for arthritics to maintain an alkaline environment? Further, they miss the connection between minerals and alkalinity. "I thought minerals were bad for me because they can become lodged in my joints thus causing me more pain," they say. Let's explore this issue further.

In the internal human environment we are mostly made up of water (60%) that flows back and forth through compartments divided by semi-permeable membranes. When all systems are "go," the body is in a state known as homeostasis—it lives and breathes to maintain this balance. However, the internal fluid of the human body works within limited tolerances of volume, acidity and electrolytes (dissolved minerals in the blood). When this balance is disrupted, as during an arthritic disturbance or other illness, the body's restorative powers begin to falter. The complex interchange of body chemicals is thrown off as the system moves toward an acid state versus its calm, neutralizing alkaline state.

To demonstrate a similar breakdown of internal systems, Dr. A. Darrell Wolfe, a twenty-year clinical nutritionist and director of the Wolfe Clinic in Nova Scotia suggests pulling the plug on your refrigerator and watching all the things (mold, bacteria, "bugs") that begin to appear and start crawling around. According to Dr. Wolfe, they were always there, but because of the original environment, they and their destructive capabilities were controlled.

Similarly, as your arthritic disturbances become more severe and occur more frequently, your pH or level of homeostasis diminishes. pH, which stands for the "potential of hydrogen," is measured on a scale of 0 to 14. Zero to six is classified as acidic, while eight to fourteen is categorized as alkaline. Seven is neutral. See figure 5.1 below.

pH SCALE

Acid												Alkaline	
Very Dangerous		Dangerous		Warning		Neutral		Warning		Dangerous		Very Dangerous	
1	2	3	4	5	6	7	8	9	10	11	12	13	14

(Figure 5.1)

Our internal systems and organs can become rigid and slowly eaten away by excessive accumulation of acid. The cells of the body are sensitive to their internal environment and cannot function in an acid environment. Diet plays an important part in maintaining a proper alkaline environment. Meats and meat by-products, as well as coffee, tea, alcohol, butter, cream, fish, grains, breads and pastas are all acid-forming foods. These foods are neutralized by the consumption of fresh fruits and vegetables.

THE MINERAL CONNECTION

While minerals can be a problem for arthritics, their proper balance in the body is critical. Minerals have a profound effect on neutralizing toxic waste matters, constructing joints and other tissues, as well as in proper immune functioning. When minerals are in balance they actually reduce, or keep in check, the toxic capabilities of their counterparts. In other words, they work in unison to keep themselves soluble so that they are utilized properly for structural purposes instead of being lodged as waste in tissue, thus causing unwanted pain.

As we consume more fruits and vegetables, we are actually building up our alkaline reserves—sort of like a bank account. These reserves are made up of minerals. Hence the need to maintain proper mineral balance.

Many alternative health practitioners today recommend the use of a liquid colloidal mineral formula. Such a formula is derived from plants that have already broken down the mineral to its smallest state, the ion. When the minerals are broken down and dissolved in the blood they form electrolytes. In this dissolved state, minerals in their electrolyte form are able to produce the electrical stimulus that keeps our hearts beating and our nerve fibers and nerve endings working. These minerals in electrolyte form actually create a healthy environment which permits other nutrients to do their work.

Mineral supplements bought over the counter have to be digested and assimilated before their health-giving properties can be realized by human tissue. This process can take anywhere from fifteen to twenty-one hours. Liquid colloidal minerals are already ionized, which means they have already been broken down, and will bypass the whole digestive process. In essence, they are ready for immediate use!

TESTING YOUR pH LEVELS AT HOME

To test your pH levels at home simply purchase some pH test strips from a drugstore or wholesale outlet. Please read directions carefully. Take a base pH reading by dropping your pH strip in a cup of your urine. Do this first thing in the morning. Record your reading, or the color code. Then, for two days eat a variety of acid-ash producing foods—like red meats, poultry, hot dogs, fast food, chicken, pork, bacon, sausage, spaghetti or other processed foods.

On the morning following your two-day food "feast" take another pH reading. If it registers on the alkaline side, your proper state of homeostasis is probably faltering. Normal pH levels are slightly acid at rising. Alkalinity at this time indicates your system has gone to a backup mode (which is not good) to neutralize what it perceives as a threat to its normal equilibrium.

More about proper pH balance and how it relates to arthritic problems can be found in Dr. Wolfe's informative and concise book, *Reclaim Your Inner Terrain*. (Copies can be purchased at: 1-800-592-9653.)

Dr. Wolfe is also involved in pioneering research with a product called "coral calcium," which has been clinically proven to be effective at reducing and preventing the negative aspects of a number of metabolic disorders like arthritis, breast cancer and prostate cancer.

THE ART OF EATING FOR THE ARTHRITIC

We need an ample supply of vegetables and fruits to neutralize the acid produced when we consume meats, fish, poultry, dairy products, seeds, nuts and grains. Also, as we age our enzyme supply starts to decline. In fact, scientific studies have shown that a sixty-year-old person in some cases can have fifty percent fewer enzymes than a thirty-year-old individual. Furthermore, data conclusively shows that aging or illness, or how we combine certain foods at mealtime, can mean the difference between good or improper digestion. And poor digestion can ignite the symptoms of arthritis. (Null, 1972; Shelton, 1994; Pizzorno, 1987; Wilson, 1994; Cheraskin, et al., 1987.)

FOOD COMBINING MADE SIMPLE

According to Dr. Ted Morter (1995) we can change our eating habits to include more of the foods that are more advantageous to us. The following chart shows how to utilize food combinations that will assist in negating, minimizing and preventing arthritic discomfort. The key to the chart is the single and double lines that separate the different food groups. Aggregates of food that are isolated by only a single line can be consumed at the same time.

For example:

- Starch foods can be eaten with vegetables and salads.
- Proteins can be combined with vegetables and salads.
- Sweet melons and fruits (separated with a double line) should be eaten alone, and not combined with other foods.

After eating, we should allow an hour or so to pass before moving to another food category. (See Figure 5.2)

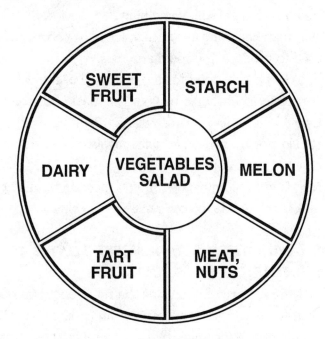

Figure 5.2.
Dr. M. Ted Morter, Jr., M.A., *Your Health Your Choice*, Hollywood, Fla.: Lifetime Books, 1995. Used with permission.

When using this guide, keep in mind that food in the outer ring can be served with any nutrient separated from it by only one line. Other general food-combining pointers to keep in mind include:

- Protein and starches require completely different digestive environments. They should not be eaten together. (So much for a steak and baked potato, a hamburger on a bun, or a bagel and creamed cheese.)
- Protein should never be eaten with sweet fruit.
- Protein and sugar is one of the worst combinations (ice cream).
- Starches and fruits should not be eaten together (strawberry shortcake).
- Melons should be eaten alone—never in combination with other food.
- Begin each meal with something raw to allow the body to start manufacturing enzymes that can be carried over and used to produce your own enzymes.
- Fruit is the ideal food for the first meal of the day.
- A protein meal should be your last meal of the day.
- Liquids, including water, dilute digestive fluids; they should not be consumed with meals. Thirst doesn't accompany well-combined meals.
- Milk is not recommended. If you must drink milk, goat's milk is preferable to cow's milk.

FOODS (AND OTHER SUBSTANCES) THAT CAN IGNITE ARTHRITIC DISTURBANCES

Not only do we need to combine the right foods, we need to know which foods can actually cause arthritic flare-ups. The list that follows is not all-inclusive, but it represents some common foods or substances that can aggravate or cause arthritic disturbances.

- Alcohol
- Artificial Dairy Foods
- Artificial Sweeteners
- Aspartame
- Bacon
- Chocolate
- Coffee
- Cola Drinks
- Dairy Foods (whole fat)
- Fast Foods
- Tobacco Smoke
- Frozen Foods
- Flour
  (refined, bleached, enriched)
- Instant Foods (all types)
- Liquor
- Luncheon Meats
- Meat (red, fatty)
- Milk (homogenized cow's milk)
- Monosodium Glutamate (MSG)
- Non-Dairy Creamers
- Salt
- Sausage
- Sugar
- TV Dinners
- White Rice
- Hot Dogs

- Hydrogenated or partially hydrogenated vegetable oils

There are a number of ways that you can test your sensitivity to these foods. One method is to simply note any arthritic discomfort after ingesting certain types or groups of foods. Pay close attention to wheat and corn—these two foodstuffs are considered to be the most aggressive symptom-causative food factors from the cereal group.

A Quick Method for Testing Any Food

The following quick pulse test can be used to check out any food in under an hour. You can do so without having to establish your normal pulse rate in advance. The requirements are that you must have eaten the test food at least once within the previous five days. You must not have smoked or taken any drugs within three days, or any stimulant such as alcohol or coffee for at least twenty-four hours. You must feel free of emotional stress, excitement, infection, heavy sunburn, or the effects of exercise. And you must be free of the effects of any environmental allergy.

You will get a stronger reaction if you last ate the test food exactly five days previously and have not eaten it since.

The test must be made on an empty stomach. Hence it is best made at breakfast time.

Begin by taking your pulse a few minutes after rising. Take it while seated.

Then eat a light meal of the test food. The amount to eat is about half the size of a regular breakfast. Eat nothing but the test food and drink nothing but pure water.

After eating wait thirty minutes and take your pulse. If after eating your pulse has risen by fifteen to twenty beats per minute over the reading before the meal, this is a fair indication of a sensitivity to that food.

Provided the requirements are always met, you can repeat this test once at breakfast time on any day. The test can help serve to confirm previous tests.

The Elimination Process

Once we have determined which foods we are sensitive to, we can then begin to restrict them or eliminate them altogether. The degree to which we decide to do this will undoubtedly depend on how severe our arthritic symptoms are after the ingestion of these specific foods. In scientific terms this is called the "elimination diet." Nan Kathryn Fuchs, Ph.D., who specializes in alternative medicine, states that the effectiveness of specialized diets in eliminating pain is surrounded by controversy. She suggests that we not enter into this debate, as in her clinical experience, eliminating certain foods and making proper food adjustments *does* work. Her advice: Go through the process for six months and be the judge of whether or not this process is beneficial for you! (Fuchs, 1985).

A Few Cases in Point

Take a look at Jane, who complained of stiffness, joint pain and a feeling of general fatigue, late in the afternoon. This occurred at least two to three times a week. After examining her activity level and diet regimen on the days she had no arthritic symptoms, compared to those of the days she had afternoon discomfort, Jane found that her affinity for certain Chinese food dishes followed by ice cream caused her arthritis to flare up.

Lauri M. Aesoph, N.D., senior editor of the *Journal of Naturopathic Medicine*, and author of *How To Eat Away Arthritis* described the case of Helen W., a forty-two-year-old rheumatoid arthritic patient who for seven years took massive amounts of aspirin along with shots of cortisone. Helen W. also had to have her knees drained of excess fluid at times, and took medication to help her sleep because of the pain she experienced.

After reviewing some information on the elimination process diet, and discovering her level of food sensitivity, Helen W's swelling and severe pain diminished. She was also able to resume normal sleep patterns without the aid of medication.

THE RIGHT DIET

In designing your new anti-arthritis diet program you might consider what Dr. Ted Morter, author of *Your Health, Your Choice*, considers to be the ideal diet. That ideal diet should consist of:

- 45% cooked fruits and vegetables
- 30% raw fruits and vegetables
- 25% grains, nuts, seeds, meat, fish, or poultry.

Based on the severity of and progression of your arthritis you may have to adjust these percentages to suit your individual biochemistry.

Supplementing your diet with various antioxidants could prove to be very beneficial in reducing the pain and inflammatory episodes of arthritis. Good wholesome food is the best way to get antioxidants. Fresh fruit and vegetables (not canned) are the most advantageous source of these powerful and dynamic substances. Dark green leafy vegetables, carrots, sweet potatoes, onions and garlic are examples of antioxidant-rich foods.

Traditional natural healing remedies for arthritis usually include a vegetable-rich diet, freshly-made raw potato juice, fresh fruits such as sour cherries, sour apples, bananas and pineapples. Raw goat's milk and grains like rice, millet and kamut are also beneficial. Doctors in European health clinics have been successful using a diet of vegetable broth supplemented with green juice mixed with carrot, red beet, and celery juice daily.

Green juices and foods are steadily gaining popularity here in the U.S. also. Traditionally, these juices are rich in chlorophyll, barley grass, wheat grass, alfalfa, and kelp (sea weed), to name a few. These energy-filled green foods contain live biologically-active enzymes, meaning they are ready to go to work for you almost immediately.

For the arthritic person this means increased energy to the system to help fuel the successful operation of vital eliminative organs. An added plus here is the fact that these green foods are loaded with vitamins, minerals, protein, and have powerful antioxidant capabilities because of their flavonoid content.

Researchers now know that a considerable amount of the pain associated with gout and other arthritic disturbances are caused by metabolic disorders and sensitivity to certain foods—in essence, foods which promote a high acidic internal environment, which severely hampers metabolic activity.

MY RECOMMENDATIONS

As a consultant to the Center for Stress, Pain and Wellness Management, and as a holistic healthcare instructor, I generally recommend the following guidelines both as a preventive, and as possible treatment measures to control arthritic disturbances:

1. **Become A Food Detective.** By becoming more aware of your individual sensitivity to various foods, you will, in essence, reduce auto-immune responses and reduce allergic flare-ups.

2. **Maintain a calorie level of 50-30-20.** By maintaining a calorie level of 50% carbohydrates 30% protein and 20% fat, you will have a gradual release of glucose (blood sugar). This will enable you to maintain a steady flow of energy, while supplying the body with moderate amounts of other nutrients for growth and repair.

3. **Increase Consumption of Fruits and Vegetables.** This will supply your body with organic sodium that it can use to keep calcium and other minerals soluble. Increased consumption of fresh fruits and vegetables will also help maintain proper pH, thus moving your system toward the alkaline side. As we have learned, internal systems function better in a non-acidic environment. Elevated pH-levels encourage or set the stage for arthritic onset and progression.

4. **Use Enzymes.** Incorporating multiple enzymes will greatly assist the digestive process and the negative complications caused by the leaky gut syndrome. Since no one enzyme has the capability to do the work of another enzyme—a protease enzyme is needed to break down protein, while a lipase enzyme will break down fat—you need an enzyme supplement that contains many of them.

Limiting yourself to a hydrochloric acid supplement, for instance, is like going to war without an army.

5. **Minimize or eliminate caffeine and alcohol.** Caffeine constricts the blood vessels while alcohol inhibits those painful uric acid crystals from being properly disposed of.

6. **Increase Your Fiber Intake.** The Surgeon General recommends an intake of twenty-five grams of fiber. Many naturopathic practitioners recommend an intake of fifty grams daily. Fiber helps keep you naturally regulated. As constipation is common to many arthritics, a good balance of fiber will reduce the chances of toxemia due to a slow removal of waste products, which can invariably find their way to weakened joints. To gauge your current fiber intake refer to the Two Minute Fiber Test found in Appendix B.

7. **Eat Your Salad Last.** By waiting to eat your salad last you will flood your system with live enzymes that will aid in the digestion process.

8. **Avoid All Fast And Processed Foods.** In a nutshell, these foods are devoid of enzymes, and are laden with fat, salt, sugars and a host of other negative nutritional factors.

The focus of our next chapter will be to give a brief overview of the various alternative modalities in the control, prevention, and treatment of arthritis. It is important to remember that what one culture calls "alternative" may be normal protocol—in some cases the primary mode of care—in other cultures throughout the world. A better term to describe these modalities, and one that is slowly growing in common usage, is "complementary."

6

ALTERNATIVES IN MANAGING ARTHRITIS

If the remedy works, if the therapy can bring
about permanent betterment or cure—then it is
the correct one, even if it happens to be contrary
to accepted thinking and endorsed conventional
practices.

—Paavo Airola, N.D.
There Is A Cure For Arthritis

In their report *Hidden Health Secrets*, Cawood and Failes
(1986, pp. 26-27) note that the Arthritis Foundation used to call
all "cures" that were not medically accepted "quack cures." Now,
however, the Arthritis Foundation is being more cautious and
refers to them as "unproven remedies."

Ray Sahelian, M.D, an internationally known physician who
represents the changing attitudes and complementary treatment
modes of today has made the following statement:

I wonder if all the efforts scientists have expended in order
to find another marketable "NSAID" had instead been
channeled towards nutritional therapies, how far ahead
medicine would have been in terms of providing adequate
and safe therapies for arthritic patients (1997, p. 15).

This same sentiment was expressed by the World Health Organization in a 1993 survey that ranked the U.S. eighteenth in overall health (*Alternative Medicine Digest*, issue 16, pp. 82-83). Although we are one of the richest countries in the world, the overall health of the general population as compared to a number of other nations, Sweden for example, shows a large disparity. According to WHO, a big reason for this paradoxical imbalance is the fact that even though other countries spend less on healthcare, a "pluralistic approach" exists—that is, an open society in which conventional and alternative therapies compete and work without reprisal or repression in the medical marketplace.

This dominant, closed approach to healthcare in the U.S. is also indicted by Andrew Weil, M.D. when he states that, ". . .allopathy (conventional medicine) as an organized enterprise is not only close minded toward alternative practices but has waged constant and often unfair war against other therapeutic systems, regarding them as competition rather than intellectual challenges" (1995, p. 119).

"ALTERNATIVE" TREATMENTS FOR ARTHRITIS IN OTHER COUNTRIES

Throughout the world, and particularly in Europe, there are many primary forms of treatment that we in the United States classify as "alternative." In many cases, diet regimens, food preferences and supplemental protocols are the reasons cited as to why our world neighbors suffer less from heart disease, cancer, diabetes, arteriosclerosis, arthritis and other chronic degenerative disorders.

Let's note a few examples:

FRANCE: French researcher Dr. Jacques Masquelier is credited with the discovery of the powerful antioxidant capabilities

106

of extracts made from pine bark and grape seeds, known as Procyanidolic Oligomers, PCO's for short. (Marketed under the trade name Pycnogenol® by Horphag Research.) Additional research has shown that PCO's are attracted to connective tissue, which help protect the glycosaminoglycans and collagen.

THE NETHERLANDS: Researchers at the University of Limburg found that by administering 120-160 mg. a day of gingko biloba that they could control intermittent claudication, the painful condition in the legs as a result of depressed circulation (Hansen, 1995).

JAPAN: While CoQ10 is becoming a highly sought after supplement in the U.S., its birth and early research is credited to the Japanese. Today, millions of Japanese people use this nutrient everyday.

Clinical trials conducted by Dr. Toru Yamagami and the American researcher Dr. Karl Folkers proved that CoQ10 could significantly lower blood pressure. Researchers at Hamamatshu University in Japan found that supplemental CoQ10 reduced the number of angina attacks in heart patients by 50% as well as neutralized the damaging effects of free-radical destruction (Folkers and Yamagami, 1980).

In addition to the above, the Japanese are in the forefront of research into the anti-arthritic and antioxidant effect of soy (Anderson et al., 1995) and green tea products (Block, 1997).

GREAT BRITAIN: In Great Britain, homeopathy has a long history of use and is a mainstay as a primary method of healthcare. In fact, a recent report in the *Daily Telegraph*, based in London, revealed that in England seventy-five percent of the patients use alternative medicine. This report also stated that the market for herbs, homeopathy and aromatherapy had doubled since 1992.

Homeopathic medicines are made from plant, animal, herbal and mineral sources. Homeopathy is based on the premise of "like cures like," where infinitesimal amounts of a substance that cause certain symptoms, can be used to relieve the same symptoms.

A recent survey of members of the AMA showed that forty-nine percent of U.S. physicians are interested in including homeopathy in their practice. Forty-five percent of the doctors surveyed, however, considered homeopathy to be a non-legitimate medical practice (*British Homeopathic Journal*, 3:97, 86:113-8).

In Great Britain one of the approaches used to assist in controlling the pain associated with arthritis is with the use of homeopathic remedies, such as bryonia and sulphur.

INDIA: While India has a long history of medicinal use of herbs, the ancient philosophical system of healing known as Ayurveda, rooted in the mind-body connection, has been largely ignored in the U.S. Recently, however, through the emerging work of Ayurvedic physician Deepak Chopra, M.D., this philosophy is being brought to the forefront.

In traditional Ayurvedic medicine, herbs such as boswellia, ginger, guggul, shilajit and turmeric are used for relief of arthritis symptoms during times of discomfort.

EUROPE AND ASIA: Although the use of glucosamine has gained national attention in the U.S. over the last two years, well-controlled clinical trials of its efficacy had been conducted throughout Europe and Asia over the last two decades. Additional research conducted in the Philippines, Thailand, and Portugal have shown that some osteoarthritis sufferers using glucosamine supplements had significant reduction in pain and symptoms within thirty days.

Because of mounting pressure from the American public this international connection is beginning to hit home. A 1996 poll conducted by the Regional Health Board in Richmond, B.C., Canada found that fifty-nine percent of Canadians use alternative medicine (*Alternative Medicine*, issue 16, 1997). Here in the U.S., data collected by John Austin, Ph.D. of the Stanford Center for Research in Disease Prevention at Stanford University found that forty percent of the American public use supplements or modalities that are considered to be "alternative" or outside normal conventional medicine (*Alternative Medicine*, 1998).

In drawing some final conclusions from his study, Dr. Austin maintains that people who use alternative measures equate these methods as being more in line with their own values, beliefs, and philosophies about life, and the role health preservation plays in it.

A December 1996 poll by the National Coalition on Health Care in Washington, D.C. showed that seventy-nine percent of respondents were highly critical of and unhappy with the current health care system in the U.S.

Responding to pressure from the public, moreover, the U.S. government has established the Office of Alternative Medicine in Washington, D.C. to conduct further research into the health benefits of many international modalities, and the use of a wide range of natural supplemental routines.

THE ALTERNATIVE FRONTIERS

While this chapter cannot cover all the past and present alternative modalities, the following synopsis reviews some that have been used with success to treat arthritic disturbances and other metabolic disturbances. At the end of this chapter you will find a list of recommended books that deal with the subjects touched upon here.

ACUPUNCTURE

This procedure stimulates endorphins, the body's natural painkillers. An acupuncturist inserts tiny needles into the body at specified pressure points along pathways known as meridians. The therapy works on the premise that blockage of vital energy along these metabolic pathways can inhibit proper function or aggravate many chronic conditions.

AROMATHERAPY

This ancient art employs the use of essential oils extracted from herbs and flowers that have scientifically shown the ability to reduce stress, alleviate pain, induce sleep, encourage proper organ function, or stimulate sexual arousal. Essential oils are applied to the skin, used in bath water, and inhaled. Scientists contend that essential oils work because our sense of smell is connected to our limbic system. According to Dr. Michael Shipley, a neurobiologist at the Cincinnati College of Medicine, the limbic region in the brain influences the workings of the entire endocrine system. This system of hormones regulates our metabolism, and a host of other metabolic cycles. For treating arthritic discomfort, aromatherapists widely recommend lavender oil.

AYURVEDIC MEDICINE

Ayurveda, a natural healing approach which has its origin over 5,000 years ago in India, is the oldest system of medicine. One of the most popular supplements to treat arthritic discomfort used by Ayurvedic practitioners is boswellia serrata. Boswellic acids have the ability to block the formation of leukotrienes. Boswellia is now available in leading vitamin stores, in extract, tablet and capsule.

BIOFEEDBACK

This non-invasive technique uses an electronic monitoring device that records information about subtle changes in body

110

functions. This information is then used to teach guided relaxation techniques that are designed to control pain and certain body functions that are directly related to stress.

BIOMAGNETIC THERAPY

This therapy dates back to 3000 B.C.E. and is recorded as part of ancient Chinese medicine. Researchers in this field theorize that by the use of the proper magnetic activity, problem areas (such as arthritic joints) can be manipulated in such a way as to encourage healing.

CHELATION THERAPY

This treatment focuses on the removal of toxic metals and minerals in the body. A solution of synthetic amino acid "EDTA" is administered intravenously. This procedure, both preventive and as a treatment, inhibits free-radical aggression. Researchers believe that by eliminating this toxic build-up, chronic metabolic disorders like arthritis and hardening of the arteries can be prevented.

COLON THERAPY

Because arthritics suffer from constipation, good colon health is essential. Alternative practitioners will recommend a healthy intake of fiber, acidophilus (friendly bacteria) and in some cases the administration of a colonic, a procedure that internally bathes the colon to remove debris from the walls.

DETOXIFICATION

Alternative practitioners use a variety of detoxification methods to maintain proper pH balance, boost immunity and rid the system of unwanted waste. It is highly recommended that arthritic patients employ daily detox routines as a preventive measure, since these methods improve flexibility, strength, energy, and lessen sensitivity to allergens. Of course, before starting any new program it is vital to check with your healthcare professional.

Some daily detox routines include:

- Epsom Salt Baths: These are suggested as a means of drawing toxins from the body. When preparing the bath make the water as hot as you can tolerate it. Add one to two pounds of Epsom salt to the bath water and soak. *Special note:* Extremely hot baths can cause fatigue. Please moderate the water temperature as it relates to your overall comfort.

- Dry Brush Massage: This method is designed to stimulate the hundred of tiny sweat glands. The skin acts much like the kidneys and serves as a valuable eliminative organ. When the skin becomes inactive and stagnant, uric acid and other toxins remain in the body.

  For the massage, purchase a coarse bath glove, a loofah mit or a coarse sponge. Brush until your skin becomes warm, using slight pressure for five to ten minutes. Once the dry brush massage is done you should shower to wash away all the dead skin and debris.

- Drink Clean, Fresh Water: Drinking at least eight glasses of water a day will help eliminate toxins and flush the kidneys.

- Apple Cider Vinegar and Honey Flush: Mix two teaspoons of raw apple cider vinegar and two teaspoonfuls of honey in a glass of water. Drink with each meal. This daily detox method is intended to mimic the actions of hydrochloric acid, the stomach acid responsible for mineral absorption, especially the absorption of calcium. Improper calcium absorption can cause arthritic disturbances. As we age our bodies produce less hydrochloric acid.

- Olive Oil Detoxification: This routine is to flush the gallbladder and stimulate bile secretion. Bile is instrumental in the breakdown of fat and helps lower blood cholesterol. Olive oil stimulates the release of bile, as well as encourages the pancreas to release bicarbonate and digestive enzymes, which help maintain an alkaline environment, and clean up excess debris that could find its way to painful arthritic joints, thus causing more pain.

At rising, before breakfast, on an empty stomach, take on ounce of olive oil with about four ounces of lemon or grapefruit juice. *Special Note:* In naturopathic circles the olive oil detox is widely known. However, for the arthritic individual, or during an acute arthritic attack, I suggest limiting or eliminating the use of lemon or grapefruit juice. These acidic juices may slow the production of the fluids that keep the joints lubricated. Rather, drink generous amounts of pineapple juice, which is rich in bromelin, the "pac-man-like" enzyme that eats up dead debris in joints. (See Alexander, 1968; and Bland, 1987.)

- Take Acidophilus: Within the intestinal tract there are hundreds of strains of bacteria. Some are more beneficial than others. Acidophilus is one of the most beneficial, as it is responsible for helping to maintain proper intestinal flora which protects the whole body from harmful bacteria. When an imbalance of gut flora occurs, tissue damage and poor circulation could result in chronic gastrointestinal inflammation, known as the leaky gut syndrome. The overgrowth of the "bad guys" (such as ancylostoma duodenale—hookworm, staphylococcus, salmonella and streptococcus) accelerates arthritic discomfort. The parasites (or "bad" bacteria) literally eat away and break down the intestinal mucosa that acts as a traffic cop that only allows essential nutrients from properly digested foods to pass through it and enter the bloodstream. Daily dosages of acidophilus are extremely useful in building that healthy bacteria. Follow manufacturer's suggested dosage range.
- Take Cleansing Herbs: There are a multitude of herbs revered for their ability to cleanse and purify the system by discouraging

the buildup of toxins. Many of these herbs, such as alfalfa, burdock root, chickweed, dandelion, fenugreek, garlic, goldenseal, milk thistle and red clover can be purchased separately or in a combination formulas. These formulas can be used on a cyclic basis, such as, taken daily for two weeks, then not taken for a week; or as part of a monthly or quarterly cleaning cycle. Many cleansing formulas can be purchased over the counter at your local health and vitamin retailer.

There are scores of daily detox protocols you can use. Some other detox methods include: fasting; massage therapy; stress reduction exercises; drinking one to two glasses of warm water after lunch or dinner; stopping cigarette smoking; increasing fiber intake, exercise, the practice of deep breathing; meditation; avoidance of processed foods and eating under stressful conditions.

LIVE JUICE THERAPY

In alternative circles the nutrients and live enzymes provided by fresh raw juices are used to treat a number of disorders. These raw juices provide nutrients that help to re-alkalinize the body's internal environment or prevent the internal environment from becoming too acidic. Dr. Norman Walker, a pioneer of live juice therapies, found in his research that one pint of carrot and celery juice daily helped rebuild and regenerate the cartilage and joints. Through the Norwalk Laboratory of Nutritional Chemistry and Scientific Research, Dr. Walker has compiled a list of combinations of various raw juices that have proven to be effective in combating the degenerative nature of arthritis, as well as other related complications (1970).

VISUALIZATION TECHNIQUES

Visualization and relaxation techniques have been used for centuries, and can be guided by a therapist's voice or a tape-recorded message. They have been beneficially used in autogenic training, biofeedback and hypnosis. Based on the concept that the mind, psychological processes and the physical body are an integrated system, visualization has had profound results in the reduction of pain and in the increase of natural healing efforts within the body. They can also be used in improving form in sports and other activities, and can aid in relaxation.

THE "HANDS-ON" APPROACH

Deep-Tissue Bodywork is a realm of treatment that focuses on the use of a number of "hands-on" techniques designed to restore myofascial function. Myofascia are the body's connective tissues that surround the muscles. Pamela Peters, Ph.D., founder and president of the Center for Stress, Pain and Wellness Management in Wilmington, Delaware employs deep-tissue bodywork with many individuals who do not respond to conventional treatments. Dr. Peters states that the object of myofascial release is to free up all restricted areas of the body. She also maintains that athletes who receive this therapy report improved muscular tone, plus increased agility and flexibility. In her clinical experience, as a treatment and preventive measure, myofascial release has proven to be very effective in reducing chronic pain and recurring ailments.

Dr. Peters cites the following cases in which deep-tissue bodywork was employed successfully:

Case 1— A seventy-year-old woman

Because the various medications to alleviate arthritic symptoms had lost their luster, a seventy-year-old woman sought alternative advice. She had trouble walking due to inflammation, and fluid build-up was making it difficult to bend and flex her knees. Dr. Peters recommended several weeks of combined therapy that included:

115

- Therapeutic Touch: used to bring balance physically, spiritually and emotionally
- Myofascial Release: to balance the hips, pelvic area, hamstrings and knees to reduce pain and swelling
- Acupressure: used on knees, hips and spine to reduce inflammation and to break up hardened tissue
- Reflexology: used on the feet to treat body mechanisms and to aid in the healing process.

Dr. Peters was successful in reducing the woman's pain level in the first treatment. After several weeks of therapy she was able to restore full range of motion in the patient's knees, and the woman was pain free, overall.

Case 2—A fifty-year-old businesswoman

This patient, diagnosed with rheumatoid arthritis, was unhappy with traditional medical treatments. She turned to homeopathic medicine but still found no relief in her symptoms.

The condition had affected both hands, knees and feet, and was diminishing her capacity to run her business, which required use of her hands and many hours of standing.

The client received therapeutic touch, myofascial release, acupressure and reflexology treatments once a week for about one year. During this time Dr. Peters stated that the patient's pain level was dramatically reduced, as was her swelling, and that movement was restored. The most important factor in this treatment protocol was the general reduction in the use of pain medication, and the eventual cessation of it.

According to Dr. Peters, numerous hands-on techniques are viable alternatives to dangerous drugs and pose little to no contraindications. Some of those therapies include:

Acupressure. This method uses the same principles and meridian points as acupuncture, but works without needles through applying specific pressure on points along the major meridians or channels of energy that run through your body. Acupressure is used to regulate, balance and normalize body function.

Craniosacral Therapy. This manual therapeutic procedure treats distortions in the structure and function of the craniosacral mechanism—the brain, spinal cord, the bones of the skull, the sacrum (the triangular-shaped bone forming the posterior wall of the pelvis), and interconnected membranes.

Massage. Massage encourages the lymphatic flow, tones muscles and stretches connective tissue.

Reflexology. There are reflex points on the feet and hands that apparently correspond to each organ, gland and structure of the body. When pressure or massage is applied to these points, reflexology improves blood supply and unblocks the functioning of nerve impulses.

Shiatsu. This approach also involves pressure on the acupuncture points to balance body energy levels, muscular, circulatory and lymphatic systems.

Therapeutic Touch. Sometimes called "laying on of hands," this method does not require contact with the body. Simply placing hands over or around the affected part is often enough to balance and bring harmony to the entire body and being.

Trager™ work. This treatment is a rhythmic technique used to re-educate the muscular structure of the body. The goal of this form of treatment is to break up sensory and mental patterns that inhibit free movement and thereby cause pain and disruption of normal function.

EXERCISE: THE FORGOTTEN TREATMENT

Exercise is important, even to the individual suffering from arthritis. In fact, the Arthritis Foundation advises those with rheumatoid or osteoarthritis to seek out qualified trainers who can guide them in exercise programs that have been formulated for arthritic patients. According to Debra Lappin, chairperson of the Arthritis Foundation, nationwide aquatic programs set up at YMCAs across the country are particularly valuable.

Robert Willix, M.D. maintains that exercise is of vital importance because the cartilage is subject to several problems because blood doesn't flow into it. Cartilage is intact, with its own fluid called synovial fluid. Synovial fluid can be compared to the oil in an automobile. Without adequate levels of oil, the parts in your engine wouldn't be able to move freely, causing the buildup of intense friction, leading to undue wear and tear of vital engine parts. Eventually, under this type of stress your car will overheat, causing a complete deterioration of vital engine parts.

For the arthritic patient who chooses not to exercise, missing "oil" in your car equates to a problem with the synovial fluid in joints. The only way to rid the synovial fluid of waste and stimulate the intake of vital nutrients is via movement of the joint. Exercise and the movement of weakened joints are therefore crucial parts of any sound program designed to manage the negative symptoms that many arthritic individuals endure.

Without proper exercise the joints build up friction like that in your car engine. The difference here, however, is that this stress on the joints causes severe pain and the proliferation of free radicals, thus invoking the auto-immune response.

The other insidious factor in this equation is weight gain. Researchers maintain that due to the sedentary lifestyles many arthritic individuals adopt, they further perpetuate this cycle of stiffness, pain, and inactivity. While studies suggest that no direct relationship exists between obesity and the development of osteoarthritis, current research has revealed that obesity clearly aggravates it.

In the past, medical experts suggested that persons with arthritis abstain from exercise to help ease and reduce joint pain, but today researchers have found that low-impact or non-impact aerobic exercise can actually improve joint motion and lessen arthritic discomfort. The most important thing to remember is that omission of this vital part of learning how to manage arthritis will eventually cause a complete breakdown of other systems. *Please check with your healthcare provider about this.*

EMPIRICISM HAS SOME VALIDATION

Empiricism is the doctrine that all knowledge is derived from sense experience. H. Curtis Wood, M.D., a very early pioneer who studied the effects of nutrition and the progression of disease, challenged the widespread condemnation of evaluation based on a patient's practical feelings or experiences. It is important to remember that how *you* feel and any consequent positive progression are strong indicators of perceived outcome and validate the course of action chosen. For example, a study by Fine and Turner (1985) on the benefits of an unconventional treatment called "flotation therapy" used a method called "rest" flotation, in which subjects floated in a shallow pool of warm water of Epsom salts. Subjects reported a reduction in the severity, reoccurrence and time span of arthritic pain. According to these researchers, flotation therapy could reduce and/or eliminate the need for pain medication.

To reiterate, as stated by Dr. Paavo Airola, N.D. in the opening remarks of this chapter:

If the remedy works, if the therapy can bring about permanent betterment or cure—then it is the correct one, even if it happens to be contrary to accepted thinking and endorsed conventional practices.

In the next chapter we will take a look at you. This is where we leave all the jargon and scientific studies. Now that you know how you can control, treat and prevent arthritic disturbances, its time to put into place an individual "action plan." In order to see or experience the sweeping changes in your health that you desire, it is imperative that you have a long-term plan with interchangeable short-term goals in place. This will enable you to better manage your arthritic problems instead of them managing you!

RECOMMENDED READING

Acupuncture
Firebrace, P. *Acupuncture–The Illustrated Guide*. New York: Harmony Books, 1987.

Acupressure
Houston, F.M. *The Healing Benefits of Acupressure*. New Canaan, Conn.: Keats Publishing, 1974.

Gach, M.R. *Acupressure Potent Points, A Guide To Self-Care For Common Aliments*. New York: Bantam Books, 1990.

Aromatherapy
Cooksley, V.L. *Aromatherapy, A Lifetime Guide To Healing With Essential Oils*. Paramus, N.J.:Prentice Hall, 1996.

Schnaubelt, K. *Advanced Aromatherapy*. Rochester, Vt.: Healing Art Press, 1995.

Ayurvedic
Chopra, D. *Ageless Body Timeless Mind*. New York: Harmony Books, 1993.

Frawley, D. *Ayurvedic Healing: A Comprehensive Guide*. Sandy, Utah: Passage Press, 1989.

Biofeedback
Basmajian, J.V., (ed.), *Biofeedback: Principles And Practice For Clinicians*, Williams and Wilkins, Baltimore, MD, 1984.

Schwartz, G.E. and J. Beatty, (editors) *Biofeedback: Theory and Research*. New York: Academic Press, 1977.

Biomagnetic Therapy
Lawrence, R., et al. *Magnet Therapy*. Rocklin, Calif.: Prima Publishing, 1998.

Null, G. *Healing with Magnets*. New York: Carroll and Graf Publishers, Inc., 1998.

Chelation Therapy
Brecher, H. and A. Brecher. *Forty Something, A Consumers Guide To Chelation Therapy.* Herndon, Va.: Health Savers Press, 1997.

Colon Therapy
Jensen, B. *Tissue Cleansing Through Bowel Management.* Escondido, Calif.: Bernard Jensen International, 1981.
Collins, J. *Colonic Irrigation.* San Francisco, Calif.: Thorsons, 1996.
Gary, R. *The Colon Health Handbook.* Reno, Nev.: Emerald Publishing, 1990.

Craniosacral Therapy
Upledger, J.E. *Your Inner Physician and You, Craniosacral Therapy and Somatoemotional Release.* Berkeley, Calif.: North Atlantic Books, 1997.

Daily Detox
Townsley, C. *Cleansing Made Simple.* Littleton, Colo.: LFH Publishing, 1997.
Wade, C. *Inner Cleansing, How To Free Yourself From Joint-Muscle-Artery-Circulation-Sludge.* Paramus, N.J.: Prentice Hall, 1992.

Exercise
Sayce, V. and I. Fraser *Exercise Can Beat Your Arthritis.* Garden City, New York: Avery Publishing Group, 1989.
Jetter, J. *Bathtub Exercise For Arthritis and Back Pain.* New York: E.P. Dutton, 1986.

Live Juice Therapy
Walker, N. *Fresh Vegetables and Fruit Juices.* Prescott, Ariz.: Norwalk Press, 1970
Kordich, J. *The Juice Man's Power of Juicing.* New York: Warner Books, 1993.

Massage
Lidell, L. *The Book of Massage.* New York: Simon and Schuster, 1984.
Shaw, P. *Massage For Pain Relief.* New York: Random House, 1996.

Reflexology
Ingham, E.D. *Stories The Feet Can Tell Thru Reflexology; Stories The Feet Have Told Thru Reflexology.* Saint Petersburg, Fla.: Ingham Publishing, 1984.
Kunz, K. and B. Kunz *Hand and Foot Reflexology: A Self-Help Guide.* St. Louis, Mo.: Fireside Books, 1992.

Therapeutic Touch
Wagner, S. *A Doctor's Guide To Therapeutic Touch.* New York: The Berkley Publishing Group, 1996.
Angelo, J. *Hands-On Healing.* Rochester, Vt.: Healing Art Press, 1997.

Trager™ Work

Alternative Medicine, The Definitive Guide. Tiburon, Calif.: Future Medicine Publishing, 1997

Note: To find out more about the Trager™ approach to healing contact The Trager™ Institute, 21 Locust Avenue, Mill Valley, CA 94941, 415-388-2688

Visualization

Epstein, G. *Healing Visualization: Creating Health Through Imagery.* New York: Bantam Books, 1989.

Achterberg, J., et al. *Rituals of Healing: Using Imagery For Health and Wellness.* New York: Bantam Books, 1994.

7

ALTERNATIVES IN MANAGING ARTHRITIS

Clearly, combating degenerative disease is no
longer the physician's battle. It is yours.
—Dr. Michael Colgan, Ph.D., CCN
Rockefeller University of New York

It is time to leave all the scientific studies behind and begin to
formulate an individual action plan. That means, it is time to set
specific goals, and define the types of activities and resources that
will be needed to reach them. Additionally, establishing timetables
with expected outcomes and a back-up plan is part of the process.
Once the plan is formulated, carrying it out and continued follow-
up to monitor progress is vital to its success. Finally, we need to
decide who will be responsible for seeing that each area of the action plan is carried out.

As Dr. Micheal Colgan has stated above, the overall responsibility is yours! Not your doctor's. And I concur with Dr. Colgan. I
found for myself that when I took an active interest, and ultimately became more assertive as a health consumer, my health began
to improve.

We accept responsibility for the establishment and management of our action plan by becoming a proactive enforcer of the steps designed to help us reach our goals. With that, however, a few questions immediately come to mind:

- How do I set up an action plan?
- How do I decide on goals?
- How long should it take to reach established goals?
- Where do I look for help?
- Should I consult my doctor?
- Am I capable of doing this?
- Do I need a partner?

Answering these questions and other pertinent information about an action plan and getting the help you need to successfully carry it out is the focus of this chapter. The first part of the chapter will be devoted to the individualized action plan, and the second part, the Arthritis Directory, will give you a listing of places, people and various organizations that are actively involved with helping individuals who suffer from arthritic disturbances, as well as those looking for ways to prevent its occurrence.

Please read one so that you can begin to manage your arthritic discomfort, instead of it managing you!

ARTHRITIC DORMANCY

As a child growing up I never understood a comment that my aunt made whenever the family got together for the holidays. While she was glad to be among us, she would always remark that she hoped that ". . .nothing would disturb Arthur today."

I knew that her son's name was not Arthur, nor was her husband's. Finally, one day, I asked her what she was talking about. She explained that Arthur was something that caused her extreme pain and discomfort, and that on such a joyous occasion she would hope that he would take a break from his mischievous work. She used the name Arthur, obviously, for her condition of arthritis.

In retrospect I realize that my aunt's goal was to keep her arthritic discomfort at bay, to enjoy the day free from pain and the overall distress that an arthritic attack can cause. The overall goal of managing and treating arthritis the natural way is not to show you how to temporarily inactivate your arthritic disturbances, but to show you how to put those disturbances to rest. That is, to achieve what is referred to as a state of *arthritic dormancy*.

The word *dormant* means a state of rest or inactivity. When you expand this definition to include the multitude of related attributes, you have a better idea of what this state of arthritic dormancy means. A state of dormancy may be characterized by: calm, cessation, easing, idleness, lessening, mildness, quiet, reduction, relaxation, relief, remission, restraint, retirement, self-containedness, stillness, stoppage, subduedness, undisturbedness.

There is mounting evidence today that arthritis is not the dreaded, incurable disease as was previously thought. In fact, with the right care, nutrition and consistent effort, researchers today have discovered ways to even reverse or slow down the debilitating aspects of this painful and destructive malady.

This management and prevention of arthritis is the goal of this book. *Managing and Preventing Arthritis* means that you can set up a plan of action that will encourage arthritic dormancy for life, so that you can begin to add some new found life to your years!

A COMPREHENSIVE ACTION PLAN

Before devising any plan of action or changing any existing prescribed routines or medication, it is advisable to discuss your individual case with your healthcare professional. To gain control of what may seem like a runaway train of pain and degeneration, maintain focus on the goal of "arthritic dormancy." That means:

1. Become familiar with the nature of your form of arthritis.
2. Formulate a supplement program that will utilize the attributes of certain supplements that focus on your need levels.
3. Test your sensitivity to certain foods and take necessary steps to exchange these foods for more supportive ones, or to eliminate these foods from your diet.
4. Establish a daily, monthly, or quarterly cycle of protocols for intestinal cleansing and detoxification.
5. Re-evaluate your present dietary regimen and begin to replace poor dietary habits, foods, and other negative lifestyle factors with more beneficial ones.
6. Start slow, but look for and seek out ways to re-establish and maintain vital energy. Successful completion of step 5 will aid greatly in accomplishing step 6.
7. Check your progress and make necessary adjustments.

Let's examine each of these steps more closely.

STEP ONE: KNOW YOUR ARTHRITIS

While there are over one hundred identified forms of arthritis, we have covered the most common ones. It is important to become familiar with the specific type you have, since this will enable you to draw up a plan of action that focuses on reducing its destructive nature. You certainly wouldn't want a carpenter coming to your home to do the job of a plumber. He or she would show up with the wrong tools, equipment and most importantly with the wrong knowledge to try to fix the problem.

STEP TWO: FORMULATING THE RIGHT SUPPLEMENT PLAN

By formulating a supplement plan that is geared toward your individual problems you stand a better chance of reaching arthritic dormancy.

While it will take some time, trial and error to set up a plan that is ideal for you, you can do this on your own, and with the help of your healthcare practitioner as necessary. The keys to a good plan are supplements or protocols that:

- meet your specific nutritional needs,
- boost your immunity,
- increase the efficiency of your digestive mechanisms, and help you maintain or re-establish vital energy.

This plan will need to address your long-term, mid-term, and short-term or occasional intervention needs. For example:

Long-Term Needs (100% of the time use)—This category of supplements would include some sort of antioxidant, multiple-vitamin and mineral, and/or supplement like chondroitin or glucosamine sulfate. Long-term needs are described below.

Mid-Term Needs (50% of the time use)—Supplements here might include things your body would need in stimulating immune function, or in providing lubricating support.

Short-Term Needs (25% of the time use)—Supplements here may be centered on helping to relieve chronic problems that occur from time to time.

Occasional Intervention Needs (5% of the time use)—Items here are used for acute symptoms. Since it is impossible to utilize every supplement on the market, supplements from this category can also serve as your reservoir for possible additions to your long-term or mid-term category of supplements.

The plans that follow are generalized and may need to be adjusted by adding or deleting certain supplements to meet your individual needs. I have found these plans to be beneficial in my own quest to maintain arthritic dormancy over the last fifteen years.

Long-Term Use:

The following formulation should be used each and every day. It is part of the 100% use category:

1. Multi-Vitamin and Mineral Formula. When choosing a formula I suggest that you find one that goes beyond the 100% of recommended daily allowances. Because of your unique nutritional needs you may want to opt for a much strong formula as cited below:

Vitamins	**Minerals**
Vitamin A — 5000 i.u.	Calcium — 100 mg.
Beta carotene — 6 mg.	Magnesium — 400 mg.
Vitamin D — 400 i.u.	Zinc — 75 mg.
Vitamin E — 200 i.u.	Copper — 2 mg.
Vitamin C — 300 i.u.	Selenium — 200 mcg.
Vitamin B-1 — 100 mg.	Iron — 10 mg.
Vitamin B-2 — 100 mg.	Chromium — 10 mg.
Vitamin B-3 — 100 mg.	Boron — 1 mg.
Vitamin B-6 — 100 mg.	Manganese 5 mg.
Vitamin B-12 — 100 mg.	Molybdenum — 100 mcg.
Folic Acid — 400 mg.	Phosphorus — 1000 mg.
Pantothenic Acid (B-5)—100 mg.	
Biotin — 100 mg.	

2. Additional supplements:
   Multiple Enzyme — take daily
   Lipoic Acid — 100 mg. three times daily
   Vitamin C — 1000-3000 mg. daily
   Chondroitin Sulfate — 500-1000 mg. daily
   Glucosamine Sulfate — 500 mg. daily
   Calcium — 500-800 mg. daily.

Special Note: In this category of 100% use for additional supplements, this protocol is not "written in stone." That is, you can change this format until you have found the right combination for you.

Mid-Term Needs:

The products here are suggestions, and as stated above can be adjusted to meet your individual needs. I have found the products below to be most beneficial. They are viable options for long-term use also. These additional supplements can be taken three to four times a week:

- Soy Isoflavones — 100 mg.
- Omega 3 Fish Oils — 1000-2000 mg.
- Vitamin E — 400-8000 i.u.
- CoQ10 — 100 mg.
- Bioflavonoids — 500-3000 mg.
- Gingko Biloba — 50-200 mg.
- Liquid Colloidal Formula — follow manufacturer's directions
- Multi-Amino-Acid Formula — follow manufacturer's directions.

Special Note: It may not be necessary to take all six of these products depending on your individual case. You may find that one or more of these mid-term products does the job for you.

Short-Term Needs:

The supplements or protocols here are designed to meet or be established as part of a cyclic routine. For example, the herbs goldenseal, burdock root, and red clover may be used as part of a three-month internal cleansing program. Or the herb milk thistle (for the liver) may be part of a monthly plan to help detoxify your liver. This program would run for two weeks, and then stop, to resume again the following month.

Special note: Please follow manufacturers guidelines when using the above products. Also, refer to the references at the end of Chapter 6 under the heading of *Detoxification* for recommended books about internal cleansing.

Occasional Intervention Needs:

These supplements are geared toward help in the elimination of pain and inflammation. Additionally, as new products are developed, you may wish to implement them for a month or two. This will give you time to evaluate how the product is working for you, and if it has merit in your case.

Some products to consider are:
- Devil's Claw, for uric acid reduction
- Dandelion, a blood purifier
- Alfalfa, for pain
- White Willow Bark, for pain
- Yucca, for pain
- Butcher's Broom, for circulation
- Arnica, for pain
- Fever Few, for inflammation
- Garlic, an antibiotic.

Special note: Please follow manufacturer's guidelines when using these products.

Step Three: Testing Your Food Sensitivity

In Chapter 5 we discussed how to test for food and substance sensitivity. With this procedure in mind realize that you have an invaluable tool for controlling or at least minimizing your arthritic flare-ups. As mentioned, you may want to keep a daily diary of your food consumption and record what your reactions were for a few months. In doing so you may be able to see a pattern forming in reference to foods that seem to precipitate acute attacks.

STEP FOUR: DETOXIFICATION PROTOCOLS

Detoxification methods are discussed at length in Chapter 6. To reiterate, I strongly suggest setting up monthly or quarterly intestinal cleansing programs. These may include: fasting, live juice therapy, colon cleansing, and many others.

In addition, there are many daily and cyclic herbal routines you can employ. It is always important here to check with your healthcare professional to decide which plan may be best suited for you. In our highly toxic society, detoxification is vital for the arthritic person to reaching and maintaining arthritic dormancy.

STEP FIVE: YOUR DIETARY REGIMEN

It is essential to set up and maintain a food program in which seventy-five percent of what you eat is fruits and vegetables. Eliminate or reduce as much as possible your consumption of red meats, dairy products, salt, sugars and alcohol. Please see Chapter 5 for a more complete coverage of this vital topic. And, stay alert for new foods to add to your dietary regimen that will help your progress.

STEP SIX: REESTABLISH VITAL ENERGY

Current data, as we have learned, shows that in many cases arthritic disturbances take years to become fully evident. Since this disease usually manifests later in life (generally after age fifty), there is a general misconception that with advancing age there is a complete breakdown in systems and a consequent loss of energy. While this is not necessarily true, it is an important consideration for all of us.

For the arthritic, maintaining energy is paramount. To do that it is imperative that you follow through on the *Seven Steps* we have been discussing. All of these factors will encourage your body to utilize its natural energy potential to fuel bodily processes, and thereby help offset the drain of energy during an arthritic attack.

STEP SEVEN: CHECK YOUR PROGRESS

Once your plan is in place mark your calendar for a date at least three months from that point, at which time you will do a realistic assessment of progress toward your goals. You need to give yourself some time for the treatments and supplements to take effect, and not change the plan after only a few days, unless it is absolutely necessary. Remember the word "flexibility." If the plan isn't working well after a reasonable period of time you can always change it.

Along the same line, do not badger yourself if you fail to follow through today or tomorrow with the goals you have set. Simply get back on course. Even if you drop your plan for a longer period of time the important thing is always to start again. This is the beauty of having a plan to follow and goals to work toward. In this way you are managing and steadily gaining control of your arthritis.

YOU ARE NOT ALONE

Many of the people I talk to feel that they are hopelessly trapped and bound by their arthritis. This is not true! However, it might be important to consider taking on a partner in the deal—that is, investing the help of a health practitioner, or becoming part of an organization or program that encourages active participation by the arthritic.

In the pages that follow you will find out where to get the help you need to meet your goals. There are literally hundreds of helpful organizations, including pain and health centers, across the country.

You now have a plan, begin to implement it. And look beyond arthritis at all the things you could and should be doing. Expand your vision and see what can be and is being done. You can move toward a greater state of health. Continue to expand your knowledge, and make the necessary changes. In the end, a new and more energetic life will emerge for you.

CONCLUSIONS

While there are many factors that can contribute to the manifestation, onset and final development of arthritis, to understand this long-term degenerative cycle, the following basic principles should always be considered:

1. Arthritis is not an unrelated, localized disease of certain joints. It is a systemic constitutional disease, that always affects the whole body.

2. Arthritis can be caused by metabolic disorders that effect and can cause pathological biochemical changes in all tissues, especially in collagen.

3. These biochemical changes can trigger inflammatory and degenerative changes in joints and their surrounding connective tissue.

4. The underlying causes for these systemic disturbances are found in prolonged abuses to which the body has been subjected. These disturbances can result from faulty nutritional patterns, overeating, nutritional deficiencies, lack of exercise, severe emotional or physical stresses.

5. The biological treatment for arthritis then should be aimed at eliminating and changing all health-destroying conditions that exist within the individual that lead to the disease.

6. The biological treatment also must seek to return to normal all metabolic processes, in essence, a rebuilding of the general overall health of the patient.

7. When the above negative factors are removed and replaced with an more appropriate health revitalizing program, the

body is strengthened and better able to initiate, utilize, and sustain its own curative powers.

Once you understand the nature of the factors that lead to the development of this malady, the more you see that to eradicate or minimize its destructive ability requires a comprehensive approach.

Think big! Believe you can make progress toward better health and you will. David Schwartz, author of *The Magic of Thinking Big* states: ". . .there is nothing magical or mystical about the power of belief." He maintains that, ". . . belief, the 'I'm positive I can' attitude, generates power, skill and energy needed to do. When you believe 'I can do it,' the how to do it develops."

Inevitably what you do or don't do will determine the intensity of your discomfort. Please remember, the U.S. Surgeon General has said that you the individual can do more for your own health and well-being than any doctor, any hospital, drug, or any exotic medical device.

Continue to cultivate your full health potential, but more importantly become an effective manager of it. It is your most precious resource.

Please get started today and take charge of your health. Remember, you are the key in turning your situation around. Good luck, and as always, Good Health to You!

THE ARTHRITIS DIRECTORY

The following lists contain many of the organizations and some of the well-known health and research centers that employ alternative methods to fight the debilitating effects of arthritis. The associations are good sources to use when looking for a particular type of practitioner, or current information on products, services and various protocols.

ASSOCIATIONS

American Academy of Allergy and Immunology
611 W. Wells Street
Milwaukee, WI 53202
(414) 272-6071

American Association of Nutritional Consultants
810 S. Buffalo Street
Warsaw, IN 46580
(888) 828-AANC

American Association of Naturopathic Physicians
2366 East Lake Avenue, East, Suite 322
Seattle, WA 98102
(206) 298-0126

American Association of Alternative Healers
PO Box 10026
Sedona, AZ 86336-8026
(520) 345-8622

American Chronic Pain Association
PO Box 850
Rocklin, CA 95677
(916) 632-0922

American College of Rheumatology
60 Executive Park Street, Suite 150
Atlanta, GA 30329
(404) 633-3777

American Foundation of Traditional Chinese Medicine
505 Beach Street
San Francisco, CA 94133
(415) 776-0502

American Holistic Medical Association
4101 Lake Boone Trail, Suite 201
Raleigh, NC 27607
(919) 787-5181

American Naturopathic and Holistic Association
3509 Connecticut Ave. N.W., Suite 565
Washington, DC, 2008-2470

American Preventive Medical Association
459 Walker Road
Great Falls, VA 22066
(703) 759-0662

Arthritis Foundation
1314 Spring Street
Atlanta, GA 30309
(404) 872-7100

Healing Alternatives Foundation
1748 Market St., Suite 205
San Francisco, CA 94114
(415) 626-4053

Health and Healing Trust P.A.
2040 Sixth Ave.
Neptune, NJ 07753
(888) 994-HEAL

Lupus Foundation of Greater
Washington
515-A East Bradock
Alexandria, VA 22314
(703) 684-2925

National Association for Human
Development
1620 Eye St., N.W. #17
Washington, DC 20006
(202) 638-3912

NIH/ National Arthritis and
Musculoskeletal and Skin
Disease Association
9000 Rockville Pike
Bethesda, MD 20892
(301) 495-4484

National Center for Homeopathy
801 North Fairfax Street, Suite 306
Alexandria, VA 22314
(703) 548-7790

Touch For Health Association
6955 Fernhill Drive,
Malibu, CA 90265
(800) 466-TFHA

HEALTH, PAIN AND RESEARCH CENTERS

The centers listed below are actively involved with the treatment of arthritic individuals as well as in designing programs that are geared toward restoring overall health.

American Whole Health Inc.
Lincoln Park Center
990 W. Fullerton Avenue Suite 300
Chicago, IL 60614
(773) 296-6700

The Center for Stress, Pain and Wellness Management Inc.
315 West 36th Street
Wilmington, DE 19802
(302) 654-1840

Duke University Medical Center
Rheumatology Clinic
P.O. Box 3892
Durham, NC 27710
(919) 684-8111

King County Natural Medicine Clinic
403 East Beker Suite 200
Kent, WA 98031
(253) 852-2866

Magaziner Medical Center
1907 Greentree Road
Cherry Hill, NJ 08034
(609) 424-8222

Mayo Clinic Pain Center
200 First Street, S.W.
Rochester, MN 55901
(507) 284-2511

National Health East
National College of Naturopathic
Medicine
11231 SE Market Street
Portland, OR 97216
(503) 255-7355

New York University Medical Center
Rusk Rehabilitation Institute
400 East 34th Street
New York, NY 10016
(212) 312-5000

Parcells Cleanse Center
P.O. Box 2129
Santa Fe, NM 87504
(800) 811-6784
or (505) 986-1441

Schachter Center for Complementary
Medicine
Two Executive Blvd Suite 202
Suffern, NY 10901-4164
(914) 368-4700

The Atkins Center for Complementary
Medicine
152 East 55th Street
New York, NY 10022
(212) 758-2110

The Corsello Centers for
Nutritional Complementary Medicine
175 East Main Street
Huntington, NY 11743
(516) 271-0222

The Integrative Medicine Clinic
The University of Arizona
College of Medicine
P.O. Box 245153
Tucson, AZ 85724-5153
(520) 694-6555

The Kaplan Clinic
5275 Lee Highway Suite 200
Arlington, VA 22207
(703) 532-4892

The Longevity Research Center
P.O. Box 12619
Marina Del Ray, CA 90295
(310) 821-2409

The New Life Health Center
12 Harris Avenue
Jamaica Plain, MA 02130
(617) 524-9551

The Ohio Pain Management Center
393 East Town Street Suite 127
Columbus, OH 43215
(614) 488-5971

The Oaks at Ojai Health Spa
122 E. Ojai Avenue
Ojai, CA 93023
(800) 753-6257

The Pain and Stress Center
5282 Medical Drive Suite 160
San Antonio, TX 78229-6023
(210) 614-7246

The Palms at Palm Springs Health Spa
572 N. Indian Canyon Drive
Palm Springs, CA 92262
(800) 753-7256

The Raj Maharishi Ayur-Veda Clinic
1734 Jasmine Avenue
Fairfield, IA 52556
(800) 248-9050

The Shealy Institute for Comprehensive
Medicine
1328 East Evergreen
Springfield, MO 65803
(417) 865-5940

The Sixth Patriarch Zen Center
2584 Martin Luther King Way
Berkeley, CA 94704, USA
(510) 486-1762
(Does personal energy analysis)

APPENDIX A

WHAT IS YOUR
ANTIOXIDANT PROFILE?

Answer each of the following questions. Then cal-
culate your score by checking the answers at
the end of this Quiz. Add them up, and
determine your Antioxidant Profile.

*1. How many servings of yellow-orange fruits and leafy green
or yellow-orange vegetables do you have daily?*
a. 2 to 4 half-cup or equivalent size servings
b. 5 to 9 half-cup or equivalent size servings
c. less than 2 half-cup servings

*2. Are the vegetables that you eat mostly fried, baked, boiled,
steamed or raw?*
a. fried
b. baked
c. boiled
d. steamed
e. raw

139

3. *Do you use "cold-pressed" vegetable oil?*

a. yes   b. no

4. *How often do you travel by airplane?*

a. more than 6 times a month

b. about 2 to 4 times a month

c. less than once a month

5. *How much time do you spend outdoors?*

a. more than 20 hours a week

b. about 5 to 20 hours a weak

c. less than 5 hours a week

6. *Do you smoke cigarettes?*

a. yes   b. no

7. *Do you have more than one or two alcoholic beverages a day?*

a. yes   b. no

8. *How close do you live to a city or an industrial manufacturing complex?*

a. live in city or near an industrial manufacturing complex

b. live in suburbs of city or several miles away from an industrial manufacturing complex

c. live in rural area, far from a city or an industrial manufacturing complex

140

9. *How often do you exercise?*

a. 3 or 4 times a week, for about 30 minutes each session

b. more than 5 times a week, each session lasting more than 30 minutes

c. less than 2 times a week

10. *Are you taking an antioxidant formula to supplement your diet?*

a. yes   b. no

YOUR *SCORE*

Below are the answers to the Antioxidant Profile Quiz. Each response is given a numeric value. A value of five is the most positive, and lower values may mean areas that need improvement Once you've finished answering the questions, tally the score to determine your Antioxidant Profile.

1. a. 2   You are not obtaining protective amounts of antioxidants from fruits and vegetables, leaving cells vulnerable to free radical destruction; eat three to five more servings a day.

    b. 5   You're getting valuable antioxidants from fruits and vegetables, especially if the vegetables are eaten raw.

    c. 0   You're not getting any antioxidants from fruits and vegetables; to help protect cells from free radical damage, eat five to nine servings a day.

2. a. 1   Frying is high in fat; heat destroys some antioxidants.

    b. 3   Baking is healthy, but usually, requires the addition of fat, and involves the loss of some antioxidants to heat.

c. 2 Antioxidants are lost through leaching and heat.

d. 4 Steaming is a healthy cooking option, but it destroys some antioxidants.

e. 5 Raw, fresh vegetables supply the most intact antioxidants.

3. a. 5 More vitamin E remains in cold-pressed vegetable oil than in oil processed with heat.

   b. 0 Certain vegetable oils are good sources of polyunsaturated fats, which are associated with helping to lower cholesterol levels. However, heat processing destroys vitamin E, increasing your need for this vitamin.

4. a. 0 Research indicates that airline passengers may be exposed to relatively high levels of radiation; the more one flies, the greater the exposure. Studies show that radiation may be associated with increased free-radical activity, increasing the need for cell-protecting antioxidants.

   b. 3 Moderate air travel exposes passengers to greater levels of radiation than if traveling by ground transportation. Even this amount of radiation exposure affects free radical activity, increasing the need for antioxidants.

   c. 5 Limited air travel lessens your exposure to elevated radiation levels associated with airline flights; therefore, your requirement for antioxidants is not affected by this activity.

5. a. 1 Excessive exposure to sunlight and ambient radiation may increase free-radical activity, possibly increasing the need for protective antioxidants.

b. 2 Moderate exposure to sunlight and ambient radiation may have an effect on free-radical activity, possibly increasing the need for protective antioxidants.

c. 5 Limited outdoor activity decreases your exposure to the harmful effects of the sun.

6. a. 0 Smoking may greatly increase the need for protective antioxidants. Vitamins E and C work synergistically to protect lung cells from free-radical activity caused by smoking.

b. 5 Yet another good reason not to smoke, as research shows that it may increase the need for antioxidants.

7. a. 0 High intakes of alcohol may greatly increase the need for all the antioxidants, particularly selenium. Moreover, all nutrients may be affected by high alcohol intake.

b. 5 Moderate to no intake of alcohol does not affect your requirement for antioxidants.

8. a. 2 Air pollution may increase your need for antioxidants.

b. 3 You may be exposed to some of the air pollution from a nearby city or industrial manufacturing plant.

c. 5 Even when living in a pollution-free environment, normal body metabolism requires antioxidants to battle free radicals.

9. a. 4 Although exercise increases your need for antioxidants, experts recommend a moderate exercise program to maintain good health. Adding a vitamin and mineral supplement insures protective amounts of antioxidants, particularly during physical stress.

143

b. 3 Excessive exercise increases your need for many nutrients, including antioxidants.

c. 5 Exercise increases the need for antioxidants. However, by not exercising regularly, you are likely to have more body fat, be overweight, and have an increased risk of associated diseases.

10. a. 5 You are assured of getting the protective amounts of antioxidants.

b. 0 You may not be getting protective amounts of antioxidants every day.

YOUR ANTIOXIDANT PROFILE

45 to 50   Excellent. You know how to live a healthy lifestyle and protect your cells with a diet rich in antioxidants—the nutrients that research shows may help to protect your body's cells from the ravaging effects of free radicals.

35 to 44   You're on the right track, but you may need to strengthen your cell-protecting antioxidant profile. Review the questions, and determine which areas need greater attention.

Less than 35   You need help! Review this quiz, and determine which areas need work. By improving your antioxidant profile, you will help prevent the destructive damage of natural body processes on cells.

TAKE THE
"2 MINUTE"
FIBER
TEST

SEE IF YOUR DAILY FIBER
INTAKE MEASURES UP
TO THE U.S. SURGEON GENERAL'S
RECOMMENDATION OF
35 GRAMS PER DAY!

Discover your daily fiber intake by choosing the foods closest to your normal daily diet for one particular day. (Note: The key to the fiber test is choosing one day's actual diet, no cheating!) Write down the grams each food provides in the space provided on the right. Add up the total to see if you are receiving the U.S. Surgeon General's recommended 35 grams of fiber per day, or the 50 to 60 grams of daily fiber recommended by many doctors, naturopaths, and nutritionists.

THE FIBER TEST:
Select only <u>ONE</u> day's actual
diet for test accuracy!

	<u>Serving size</u>	<u>Grams</u>	<u>Fiber Intake</u>
Meat	any amount	0	_____
Chicken	"	0	_____
Fish	"	0	_____
Eggs	"	0	_____
Dairy (cheese, milk, etc.)		0	_____

Grains & Pastas:

Brown rice	1/2 cup	2.4	_____
White rice	1/2 cup	0.8	_____
Spaghetti	1/2 cup	2.0	_____
Couscous	1/2 cup	0.5	_____
Millet	1/2 cup	3.5	_____
Polenta	1/2 cup	2.0	_____
Quinoa	1/2 cup	5.0	_____
Tabouli	2/3 cup	1.0	_____
Tofu	1/5 block	1.0	_____
Tempeh	1/3 block	8.0	_____

Cold & Hot Cereals:

Oatmeal	1/2 cup	7.7	_____
Grape Nuts	I oz.	1.8	_____
Wheaties	1 cup	2.6	_____
Multigrain	2/3 cup	4.0	_____
Millet Rice	3/4 cup	3.0	_____
Corn Flakes	3/4 cup	2.7	_____
Puffed Rice	1 cup	1.0	_____

	<u>Serving size</u>	<u>Grams</u>	<u>Fiber Intake</u>
Breads:			
Bagel	1	0.6	_____
Bran muffin	1	2.5	_____
Rye bread	I slice	0.9	_____
Wheat bread	I slice	1.4	_____
Multigrain	1 slice	2.0	_____
Spelt	I slice	0.9	_____
Focaccia	I slice	1.0	_____
Wheat tortilla	I tortilla	2.0	_____
White tortilla	I tortilla	0.5	_____
Beans, Peas, Legumes:			
Lentils	1/2 cup	3.7	_____
Pinto beans	1/2 cup	2.5	_____
Split peas	1/2 cup	2.5	_____
Kidney beans	1/2 cup	5.8	_____
Lima beans	1/2 cup	4.4	_____
Green beans	1/2 cup	2.1	_____
Chickpeas	1/2 cup	6.0	_____
Vegetables:			
Asparagus	1/2 cup	1.0	_____
Artichoke	1 large	4.5	_____
Romaine lettuce	1 cup	2.0	_____
Carrots	1 med.	1.5	_____
Cucumber	1/2 cup	0.4	_____
Broccoli	1/2 cup	2.2	_____
Cauliflower	1/2 cup	1.0	_____
Tomato	1 med.	1.5	_____
Potato (w/skin)	1 med.	2.5	_____
Zucchini	1/2 cup	1.8	_____
Mushrooms	1/2 cup	1.5	_____

	Serving size	Grams	Fiber Intake
Avocado	1/2	2.8	_____
Corn on the Cob	1 med.	5.0	_____
Spinach	1/2 cup	7.0	_____
Beets	1/2 cup	2.5	_____
Steamed veggies	1 large plate	6.5	_____
Tomato Sauce	1/2 cup	2.0	_____
Salsa	2 tbsp.	1.0	_____
Sea Nori	1 sheet	1.0	_____

Fruits:

Apple (w/skin)	1 med.	3.5	_____
Grapefruit	1/2	0.8	_____
Banana	1 med.	2.4	_____
Cantaloupe	1/4 melon	1.0	_____
Orange	1 med.	2.6	_____
Prunes	3	3.0	_____
Figs	1 med.	2.0	_____
Raspberries	1/2 cup	4.6	_____
Watermelon	1 slice	2.8	_____

Nuts and Seeds:

Almonds	10 nuts	1.1	_____
Peanut butter	2 tbsp.	2.0	_____
Sesame butter	2 tbsp.	2.0	_____
Sunflower seeds	1 cup	2.0	_____

Other:

Popcorn	1 cup	1.0	_____
Corn tortilla chips	1 oz.	2.0	_____
Potato chips	1 oz.	1.0	_____
Wheat crackers	4	1.0	_____
Multi-grain waffle	1	2.0	_____

	Serving size	**Grams**	**Fiber Intake**
Gardenburger	1 patty	5.0	_____

A. SURGEON GENERAL'S RECOMMENDED DAILY FIBER INTAKE: <u>35 GRAMS</u>

B. MANY DOCTOR'S, NATUROPATHS AND NUTRITIONISTS RECOMMEND: <u>50 GRAMS</u>

C. ADD UP YOUR TOTAL FIBER INTAKE FOR ONE PARTICULAR

    DAY AND INSERT: _____

D. TO SEE THE # OF ADDITIONAL FIBER GRAMS YOU NEED TO MEET THE

    SURGEON GENERAL'S RECOMMENDATOIONS SUBTRACT LINE C FROM A: _____

E. TO SEE THE # OF ADDITIONAL FIBER GRAMS YOU NEED TO MEET MANY

    DOCTOR'S RECOMMENDATIONS, SUBTRACT LINE C FROM B: _____

REFERENCES

Adams, R. and Murray, F. *Improving Your Health with Niacin (Vitamin B3)*. New York: Larchmont Books, 1978.

Aesoph, L.M. *How To Eat Away Arthritis*. Englewood Cliffs, N.J.: Prentice Hall, 1996.

Ahmad, N., et al. "Green Tea Constituent Epigallocatechin-3-Gallate and Induction of Apoptosis and Cell Cycle Arrest in Human Carcinoma Cells." *Journal of National Cancer Institute*, 1997, 89 (24): 1881-1886.

Airola, P. *How to Get Well*. Phoenix, Ariz.: Health Plus Publishers, 1987.

Airola, P. *The Miracle of Garlic*. Phoenix, Ariz.: Health Plus Publishers, 1978.

Airola, P. *There Is a Cure for Arthritis*. West Nyack, N.Y.: Parker Publishing Inc., 1968.

Albertazzi, P., et al. "The Effects of Dietary Soy Supplements on Hot Flashes," *Obstet. Gynecol.*, 1998, 91:6-11.

Alexander, D.D. *Arthritis and Common Sense*. Hartford, Conn.: Witkower Press, 1968.

Alternative Medicine Digest. "Check Your Nutrient Status with Vitamin Test." Tiburon, Calif., Issue 19, 10:97:63.

Alternative Medicine Digest. "How's Your Nutritional Status: Home Test Gives You A Quick Answer," Tiburon, Calif., Issue 24, 6:98:65-67.

Alternative Medicine Digest. "The Politics of Medicine: 31% of Americans Left Out in the Cold, Despite $1 Trillion for U.S. Health Care," Tiburon, Calif., Issue 16: 82-83.

Alternative Medicine Digest, "An Herbal Aid for Arthritis and Inflammation," Issue 24, Tiburon, Calif., June/July, 1998: 67-68.

Anderson, J.W., et al. "Meta-Analysis of the Effects of Soy Protein Intake On Serum-lipids," *New England Journal of Medicine*, 1995, 333:276-282.

Aquino, R., et al. "Plant Metabolites, New Compounds and Anti-Inflammatory Activity of Uncaria to Mentosa," *Journal of Natural Products*, Vol. 54; No.2, March-April 1991, pp. 453-459.

Aquino, R., et al. "New Polyhydroxylated Triterpenes from Uncaria to Mentosa," *Journal of Natural Products*; Vol. 53 No. 3 (May-June 1990), pp. 559-564.

Artemov, N.M. "The Biological Basis of the Therapeutic Use of Bee Venom," Dept. of Physiology and Medicine, National University of Gorki, U.S.S.R., 1959.

Arthritis Foundation. "Arthritis Foundation Warns of Future Epidemic: Center For Disease Control Issues New Report On Arthritis," *News From the Arthritis Foundation.* Atlanta, Ga., 6:23:94.

Babal, K. "Cetyl Myristoleate," *Natural Food Retailer*, New Brunswick, N.J., August/September, 1997.

Balch, J.F. and P.A. Balch *Prescription for Nutritional Healing*. Garden City Park, N.Y.: Avery Publishing, 1993.

Barton-Wright, E.C., and W.A. Elliot "The Pantothenic Acid Metabolism of Rheumatoid Arthritis." *Lancet*, October 26, 1963, pp. 862-863.

Basu, T.K., et al. "Ascorbic Acid Therapy for the Relief of Bone Pain in Paget's Disease," *Acta Vitaminologica et Enzymologica*, 32: 1-4, 45-49, 1978.

Bauer, C. *Acupressure for Everybody*. New York: Henry Holt, 1989.

Berger, P., et al. "Health, Lifestyle and Environment," New York: The Social Affairs Unit, Manhattan Institute, 1991, p. 9.

Berger, S. M., M.D. *Forever Young*. New York: William Morrow and Co., Inc., 1989.

Beyond Vitamins, The Carotenoids Come of Age. LaGrange Ill.: Henkel Corporation, 1995.

Bieler, H.G. *Food Is Your Best Medicine*. New York: Random House, 1968.

Bland, J. *Intestinal Toxicity and Inner Cleansing*. New Canaan, Conn.: Keats Publishing, 1987.

Bland, J. *Octacosanol, Carnitine, and Other "Accessory" Nutrients*. New Canaan, Conn., Keats Publishing, 1982.

Block, G. "Vitamin C and Cancer Prevention: The Epidemiologic Evidence," *American Journal of Clinical Nutrition*, 53 (1991): 2705-2825.

Block, M.A. *No More Ritalin: Treating ADHD Without Drugs*. New York: Kensington Publishing Corp., 1996.

Block, W. "Ginkgo Biloba: The World's Oldest Anti-Aging Secret," *Life Enhancement News*, Petaluma, Calif., Issue No. 28, 12:96:1-7.

Block, W. "Ancient Health Secret of the Orient, Green Tea Extract." *Life Enhancement*, Petaluma, Calif.: 9:97:3-7.

Braly, J. *Food Allergy and Nutrition Review*. New Canaan, Ct.: Keats Publishing, 1992.

Brandt, K.D. "Effects of Non-steroidal Anti-inflammatory Drugs on Chrondrocyte Metabolism In Vitro and In Vivo," *American Journal of Medicine*, 1987, (5A): 29-34.

Brewer, E.J. and K.C. Angel *The Arthritis Source Book*. Chicago, Ill.: Contemporary Books, 1993.

Broadhurst, C.L. "Season's Wheezing, Soothing Allergies with Herbs," *Herbs for Health*, Golden, Colo., May-June, 1998, pp. 54-56.

Cameron, E. and A. Campbell "The Orthomolecular Treatment of Cancer. Clinical Trail of High-Dose Ascorbic Supplements in Advanced Human Cancer," *Chem. Biol. Interacts*, 1974; 9:285-315.

Caron, J., et al. "Chondroprotective Effect of Intraacticular Injections of Interleukin-1 Receptor Antagonist in Experimental Osteoarthritis," *Arth. and Rheum.* 1996, 39:1535-1544.

Carotenoids: Information and Facts. LaGrange, Ill.: The Henkel Corporation, 1995.

Casaril, M., et al. "Decreased Activity of Liver Glutathione Peroxidase in Human Hepatocellular Carcinoma," *European Journal of Cancer Clinical Oncology*, 1985, 21:941-944.

Cassidy, A., et al. "Biological Effects of a Diet of Soy Protein Rich in Isoflavones on the Menstrual Cycle of Premenopausal Women," *American Journal of Clinical Nutrition*, 1994, 60: 333-40.

Castleman, M. *The Healing Herbs, (Ginkgo).* Emmaus, Pa.: Rodale Press, 1991.

Cawood, F.W. and J.M. Failes *Hidden Health Secrets.* Peachtree City, Ga: FC and A Publishing, 1986.

Challem, J. "CoQ10, May be the 90's Miracle Nutrient," *Let's Live*, Los Angeles: 9:95:18-22.

Challem, J. "MSM, The Newest Arthritis Cure," *Let's Live*, Los Angeles: 6:98:48-51.

Challem, J. "Vitamin C: The Master Nutrient Keeps Your Health on an Even Keel," *Let's Live*, Los Angeles: 1995: 15-18.

Cheraskin, E., and W.M. Ringsdorf et al. *Diet and Disease.* New Canaan, Conn.: Keats Publishing, 1987.

Cheraskin, E. and W.M. Ringsdorf et al. *The Vitamin C Connection, Getting Well and Staying Well with Vitamin C.* New York: Harper and Row Publishers, 1983.

Cheraskin, E. and W.M. Ringsdorf *Psychodietetics.* New York: Bantam Books, 1974.

Cichoke, A.J. "Ayurveda: The Ancient Healing System of India," *Health Food Business*, Melville, NY, 3:95; 49-50.

Cichoke, A.J. "Healing Powers of Aged Garlic Extract," *Townsend Newletter for Doctors*, 6:94.

Clark, L. *Know Your Nutrition.* New Canaan, Conn.: Keats Publishing, 1973.

Cloutatre, D. *Anti-Fat Nutrients.* San Francisco, Calif.: Pax Publishing, 1997.

Cochran, C. *Dr. Chuck Cochran Discusses Arthritis and Cetyl Myristoleate.* New York: Healing Wisdom Publications, 1997.

Colgan, M. *Your Personal Vitamin Profile.* New York: Quill, 1982.

Coronary Drug Project Research Group, "Clofibrate and Niacin in Coronary Heart Disease," *Journal of American Medical Association*, 1975, 231(4):360-381.

Cowley, G., et al. "The Vitamin Revolution," *Newsweek*, June 7, 1993.

Crain, L. *Magic Vitamins and Organic Foods.* Los Angeles: Crandrich Studios, 1976.

Crary, E. *Second International Symposium on Selenium in Biology and Medicine*, Texas Tech University, Lubbock, Texas, May, 1980.

Crayhoh, R. "Energy Therapy," *Total Health*, Vol. 20 No.1, St. George, Utah, 1998, p.14-15.

Darlington, L.C. and N.W. Ramsey "Diets For Rheumatoid Arthritis," *Lancet*, 338:1209; 1991.

DeSilva, D.M. "An Angiogenesis Primer," *International Journal of Anti-Aging Medicine*, Vol. 1. No. 1., Huntington, NY, 1998, p. 14-15.

DiCyean, E. *Vitamins and Your Life and the Micronutrients*. New York: Simon and Schuster, 1972.

Dressler, D. "Homeostasis, the Balanced State," in: *Nursing Skill Book*. Horsham, Pa.: Intermed Comm., 1979, p. 15-28.

Dunne, L.J. *Nutrition Almanac*. Third Edition, New York: McGraw-Hill,1990.

Dyerberg, J.H. and O. Bang, et al. "Eicosapentaeoioc Acid and Prevention of Thrombosis and Atherosclerosis," *Lancet,* 1978, 2:117-119.

Eaton, K.K., et al. "Gut Permeability Measured by Polyethylene Glycol Absorption in Abnormal Gut Fermentation as Compared with Food Intolerance." *Journal of the Royal Society of Medicine*, 88: 63-66; 1995.

Eisenberg, D.M., et al. "Unconventional Medicine in the United States," *The New England Journal of Medicine,* 1993; 328:246-52.

Estrada, D.E., et al. "Stimulation of Glucose Uptake by the Natural Co-Enzyme Alpha Lipoic Acid: Participation of Elements of the Insulin Signaling Pathway," *Diabetes*, 45:1798-1804; 3:96.

Gadd, I. and L. Gadd *Arthritis Alternatives*. New York: Facts on File, 1985.

"FDA Responds to Supplement Commission Report," *The Vitamin Retailer, Supplement Industry News*, East Brunswick, N.J., 6:98:14-24.

Fine, T. and J.W. Turner "Rest-Assisted Relaxation and Chronic Pain," *Health and Clinical Psychology*, 1985.

Finnegan, M. "Freedom of Movement," *The Energy Times*, Long Beach, Calif., March/April, 1995, pp. 50-54.

Fischer-Rizzi, S. *Complete Aromatherapy Handbook, Essential Oils for Radiant Health*. New York: Sterling Publishing, 1990.

Folkers, K. and T. Yamagami. *Biomedical and Clinical Aspects of Coenzyme Q*. Vol. 2, Amsterdam: Elsevier/ North Holland Biomedical Press, 1980, pp. 333-347.

Foreman, J.C. "Mast Cells and the Actions of Flavonoids," *Journal of Allergy and Clinical Immunology*, 127:546-550, 1984.

Foster, S. *Herbs for Your Health*. Loveland, Colo.: Interweave Press, 1996.

Fotsis, T., et al. "Genistein, a Dietary Derived Inhibitor of In Vitro Angiogenesis," *Proceedings of the National Academy of Sciences*, 90:3:93:2690-94.

Fox, A. and B. Fox *Immune for Life*, Rocklin, Calif.: Prima Publishing, 1990.

Fredericks, C. *Nutrition Guide for the Prevention and Cure of Common Ailments and Diseases*. New York: Simon and Schuster, 1982.

Fredericks, C. *Arthritis: Don't Learn To Live With It*. New York: Putnam, 1985.

Fuchs, N.K. *The Nutrition Detective*. Los Angeles: Jeremy Tarcher, 1985.

Fulcher, K.Y. and P.D. White "Randomised Control Trail of Graded Exercise in Patients With the Chronic Fatigue Syndrome," *British Journal of Medicine*, 1997; 314:1647-1652.

Garrison, R. and E. Sumer *The Nutrition Desk Reference* New Canaan, Conn.: Keats Publishing, 1995.

Geslewitz, G. "Attention Deficit Disorder: Rejecting the Medicated Life," *Health Food Business*, Elizabeth, N.J., 3:98:32-40.

Goldenberg, D.L. "Fibromyalgia Syndrome," *Journal of the American Medical Association*, 257 (1987): 2782-2787.

Goldin, R. H., et al. "Clinical and Radiological Survey of the Incidence of Osteoarthritis Among Obese Patients," *Annal Rheum Dis*, 1976, 35:359-363.

Gorner, P. and R. Kotulak "Scientists Try to Tame Molecular Sharks," *Chicago Tribune*, 12:11:91.

Gottlieb, B. *New Choices in Natural Healing*. Emmaus, Penn.: Rodale Press Inc., 1995.

Graham, J. *Evening Primrose Oil*. New York: Thomsons Publishers, 1984.

"Green Waves of Barley Ease Arthritis For Some," *Better Nutrition for Today's Living,* Atlanta, Ga., 9:95:42.

Guyton, A.C. *Functions of the Human Body*. Philadelphia, Pa.: W.B. Sanders, 1969.

Hansen, C. *Grape Seed Extract: The Most Potent Preventive Medicine You Can Take*. New York: Healing Wisdom Publications, 1995.

Harkcom, T.M., et al. "Therapeutic Value of Gradual Aerobic Exercise Training in Rheumatoid Arthritis," *Arthritis Rheum.*, 1985; 28:32-39.

Hatfield, F.C. and M. Zucker *Relieving Pain Nutritionally*. Woodland Hills, Calif.: Weider Health and Fitness, 1990.

Hendler, S.S. *The Complete Guide to Anti-Aging Nutrients*. New York: Simon and Schuster, 1985.

Hemrich, K. "Detox Your System," *Fit Magazine*, New York, Sept/Oct. 1997, p. 68-71.

Hennig, B. and M. Stuart "Nutrients That May Protect Against Atherosclerotic Lesion Formation," *Journal of Applied Nutrition*, Vol. 40. No. 1., 1988.

Hoffer, A. "Treatment of Arthritis by Nicotinic Acid and Nicotinamide," *Canadian Medical Association Journal*, 1959, 81, pp. 235-239.

Hoffer, A. and A. Walker *Ortho-molecular Nutrition*. New Canaan, Conn.: Keats Publishing, 1978.

Hoffman, C., et al. "Persons with Chronic Conditions," *The Journal of the American Medical Association*, 276 (10:13:96) 1473-1479.

Hoffman, R.L. *The Natural Approach to Attention Deficit Disorder (ADD)*. New Canaan, Conn.: Keats Publishing, 1997.

Howell, E. *Enzyme Nutrition*. Wayne, N.J.: Avery Publishing Group, Inc., 1985.

Huang, M.T. "Superphytochemicals," *The Energy Times*, Long Beach Calif., March/April, 1995.

Jensen, B. *The Science and Practice of Iridology*. Escondido, Calif., 1952.

Johnston, C. et al. "Antihistamine Effect of Supplemental Ascorbic Acid and Neutrophil Chemoaxis," *Journal of American College of Nutrition*, 1992; 11:172-176.

Julius, M. et al. "Glutathione and Morbidity in a Community Based Sample of Elderly," *Journal of Clinical Epidemiology* 47, No. 9 (1994): 1021-1026.

Kaufman, W. *The Common Form of Joint Dysfunction: Its Incidence and Treatment.* Brattleboro, Vt.: E.L. Hildreth Co., 1949.

Keough, C. *Natural Relief for Arthritis.* Emmaus, Pa.: Rodale Press, 1983.

Knight, J. "Reading the Leaves; Green Tea Provides Clues to Preventing Cancer, Heart Disease and More," *Herbs for Health*, Golden, Colo., May-June, 1988, pp.41-45.

Knowles, J.H. *Doing Better and Feeling Worse: Health in the United States.* New York: W.W. Norton and Company, Inc., 1977.

Krakauer, K., et al. "Postaglandin E1 Treatment of NZB/W Mice," *Clinical Immunology Immunopathology*, II (1978), pp. 256-62.

Kremer, J.M., et al. "Fish Oil Fatty Acid Supplementation in Active Rheumatoid Arthritis," *JAMA*, 1987, 258:962.

Kremer, J. "Effects of Modulation of Inflammatory and Immune Parameters in Patients with Rheumatic and Inflammatory disease Receiving Dietary Supplement of N-3 and N-6 Fatty Acids," *Lipids,* 1996.

Kronhausen, E., et al. *Formula for Life, the Anti-Oxidant Free-Radical Detoxification Program.* New York: William Morrow, 1989.

Kroner, J., et al. "The Treatment of Rheumatoid Arthritis with an Injectable Form of Bee Venom," *Annals of Internal Medicine*, 2 (7): 1077-1088 (1938).

Kulvinskas, V. *Survival Into the 21st Century.* Woodstock Valley, Conn. (P.O. Box 64, 06282): 21st Century Publications, 1975.

Kushner, I.(editor) *Understanding Arthritis, The Arthritis Foundation.* New York: Charles Scribner's Sons, 1984.

Lane, W. and L. Comac *Sharks Don't Get Cancer.* Garden City Park, New York: Avery Publishing, 1992.

LaPatra, J. *Healing, The Coming Revolution in Holistic Medicine.* New York: McGraw-Hill, 1978.

Lassen, K.O. and M. Horder "Selenium Status and the Effects of Organic and Inorganic Selenium Supplementation in a Group of Elderly People in Denmark," *Scandinavian Journal of Clinical Laboratory Investigation*, 1994; 54:585-590.

Lau, B.H.S. "Detoxifying, Radioprotective and Phagocyte-Enhancing Effects of Garlic," *Inter. Clin. Nutr. Rev.*, 9:27-31, 1989.

Levin, M. "New Concepts in the Biology and Biochemistry of Ascorbic Acid," *New England Journal of Medicine*, 314:892-902, 1986.

Leviton, R. "Reviving the Thyroid," *Alternative Medicine Digest,* 1998.

Lieberman, S. and N., Bruning *Design Your Own Vitamin and Mineral Program.* Garden City, New York: Doubleday and Company, Inc., 1987.

Lieberman, S. and N. Bruning *The Real Vitamin and Mineral Book.* New Canaan, Conn.: Avery Publishing, 1997.

Lin, R.I. "Anti-Oxidant, Pro-Oxidant, Anti-Free Radical and Radiation Protection on the Health Significance of Garlic and Garlic Constituents," *Abstract of the First World Congress on the Health Significance of Garlic and Garlic Constituents,* 1990, p.22.

Long, J.W. *Prescription Drugs.* New York: Harper and Row, 1985.

Loprinizi, C.L. "Capsicum Cream Eases Pain," *Journal of Clinical Oncology,* 1997; 15:2, 974-80.

Machlin, L. and H.E. Sauberlich "Beyond Deficiency: New Views on the Function and Health Effects of Vitamins," *The New York Academy of Sciences,* 2:92-9-12.

Madrid, F.F. *Treating Arthritis, Medicine, Myth, and Magic.* New York: Insight Books, Plenum Press, 1989.

Malone, F. *Bees Don't Get Arthritis.* New York: E.P. Dutton, 1979.

Martinez, J.E., et al. "Fibromyalgia Versus Rheumatoid Arthritis: A longitudinal comparison of the quality of life," *Journal of Rheumatology,* 1995, Feb. 22(2):270-274.

Masoro, E.J. "Biology of Aging, Current State of Knowledge," *Archives of Internal Medicine,* 147; 1987, pp. 166-169.

McCully, K.S. *The Homocystein Revolution.* New Canaan, Conn.: Keats Publishing, 1997.

McIlwain, H.H. and D.F. Bruce *The Fibromyalgia Handbook.* New York: Henry Holt, 1996.

McIlwain, H.H and B. Fulghum *Stop Osteo-Arthritis Now!* New York: Simon and Schuster, 1996, pp. 12-14.

McLeod, D.W., et al. "Investigations of Harpagophytum Procumbens A.K.A. Devil's Claw, in the Treatment of Experimental Inflammation and Arthritis in the Rat," *British Journal of Pharmacology,* 1979, pp. 104P-141P.

Memmler, R.L., et al. *The Human Body in Health and Disease.* Philadelphia, Pa.: Lippincott, 1996.

Mills, A.S. *Allergy: Facts and Fiction.* Chicago: Budlong Press, 1983.

Mindell, E. *Earl Mindell's Herb Bible.* New York: Simon and Schuster, 1992.

Mindell, E. *Earl Mindell's Soy Miracle.* New York: Simon and Schuster, 1995.

Mindell, E. "The Joy of Soy," *Herbs for Health,* Vol. 3, No. 3, Golden, Colo.: Herb Companion Press, July/Aug., 1998.

Mindell, E. *Live Longer and Feel Better with Vitamins and Minerals.* New Canaan, Conn.: Keats Publishing, 1994.

Mindell, E. *What You Should Know About the Super Antioxidant Miracle.* New Canaan, Conn.: Keats Publishing, 1996.

Moldofsky, H.D., et al. "Musculoskeletal Symptoms and Non-REM Sleep Disturbance in Patients with 'Fibrositis Syndrome' and Healthy Subjects," *Psychosomatic Medicine* 1975; 37:341.

Morales, A., et al. "Effects of Replacement Dose of DHEA in Men and Women of Advancing Age," *Journal of Clinical Endocrinological Metabolism,* 78: (360-1367), 1994.

Morgan, B.L.G. and R. Morgan *Hormones.* Los Angeles: The Body Press, 1989.

Morter, M.T. *Your Health Your Choice.* Hollywood, Fla.: Lifetime Books, 1995.

Murray, M.T. *Natural Alternatives to Over-the-Counter and Prescription Drugs.* New York: William Morrow and Co, 1994.

Murray, M.T. and J. Pizzorno *The Encyclopedia of Natural Medicine.* Rocklin, Calif.: Prima Publishing, 1991.

Murray, M.T. *Seven Valuable Tips for Managing Osteoarthritis.* Issaquah, Wash.: Vital Communications, Inc., 1998.

Naruszewicz, M., et al. "Thiolation of Low-Density Lipoprotein by Homocysteine Thiolactone Causes Increased Aggregation and Altered Interaction With Cultured Macrophages." *Nutrition, Metabolism and Cardiovascular Disease.* 4:70-77, 1994.

Naturopathic Handbook of Herbal Formulas. Ayer, Mass.: Herbal Research Publications, 1995.

Newman, N.M. and R.S.M. Ling, "Acetabular Bone Destruction Related To Non-Steroidal and Anti-Inflammatory Drugs," *Lancet,* ii: 11-13, 1985.

Norden, M.J. *Beyond Prozac.* New York: Harper Collins Publishers, 1995.

Null, G. and S. Null. *The Complete Encyclopedia of Natural Healing,* New York: Kensington Books, 1998.

Olshevsky, M. et al. *The Manual of Natural Therapy* New York: Facts on File, 1989.

Olszewski, A.J. and K.S. McCully "Homocysteine Metabolism and Oxidative Modification of Proteins and Lipids," *Free Radical Biology and Medicine,* 14:683-693, 1993.

Packer, L. and H.J. Tritischler "Alpha-Lipoic Acid: The Metabolic Antioxidant," *Free Radical Biol. Med.* 20:625-626, 1996.

Parham, B. *What's Wrong with Meat.* Denver Colo.: Ananda Marga Publications, 1979.

Passwater, R.A. *Lipoic Acid: The Metabolic Antioxidant.* New Canaan, Conn.: Keats Publishing, 1995.

Passwater, R.A. "Measuring Your Antioxidant Status: An Interview With Dr. Charles A. Thomas," *Whole Foods,* South Plainfield, N.J., 6:95-50-54.

Passwater, R.A. *Selenium as Food and Medicine.* New Canaan, Conn.: Keats Publishing, 1980.

Passwater, R.A. *The Antioxidants.* New Canaan, Conn.: Keats Publishing, 1985.

Pauling, L. *How to Live Longer and Feel Better.* New York: W.H. Freeman and Co., 1986.

Pearson, D. and S. Shaw *Life Extension.* New York: Warner Books, 1982.

Peters, Pamela, Ph.D. *Personal Interview,* The Center for Stress Pain and Wellness Management, Inc., Wilmington, Del., 6:98.

Petersdorf, R., et al. *Principles of Internal Medicine.* New York: McGraw Hill, 1983, pp. 517-24.

Pickles, H. *Pagosid Procumbens or Devil's Claw, The Remarkable Medicinal Properties.* Lynden, Wash.: Flora, Inc., 1994.

Pisetsky, D.S. *The Duke University Medical Center Book of Arthritis.* New York: Fawcett Columbine Books, 1991.

Pizzorna, J. and M. Murray *A Textbook of Natural Medicine.* Seattle, Wash.: John Bastyr College Publications, 1987.

Price, R.K., et al. "Estimating the Presence of Chronic Fatigue Syndrome in the Community," *Public Health Reports*, 107 (Sept-Oct 1992): 514-522.

Quillin, P. *Healing Nutrients*. Chicago, Ill.: Contemporary Books, 1987.

Rogers, S.A. "One of the Best Kept Secrets in Medicine: Osteoarthritis is Reparable," *Let's Live*, Los Angeles, Calif., 10:95:96.

Rogers, S. *Wellness Against All Odds*. Syracuse, N.Y.: Prestige Publishing, 1992.

Safyh, H. and E.R. Sailor "Amnon HPT-5-lipoxgenase inhibition by acety-11-keto-B-Boswellic Acid," *Photomedicine*, 1996, 3:71-72.

Salmi, H.A., et al. "Effect of Silymarin on Chemical Function and Morphological Alternations of the Liver," *Scandinavian Journal of Gastroenterolog,y* 17 (1982): 517-521.

Santillo, H. *Food Enzymes: The Missing Link to Radiant Health*. Prescott, Ariz.: Hohm Press, 1987.

Sahelian, R. *Glucosamine, Nature's Arthritis Remedy*. Marina Del Ray, Calif.: Longevity Research Center, Inc., 1997.

Schechtner, S. "Arthritis: Natural Therapies," *Health Food Business*, PTN Publishing, Melville, N.Y., 9:95:75-76.

Scheer, J.F. "Bee Propolis," *Better Nutrition for Today's Living*, Atlanta, Ga., 10:93:34-37.

"Sea Cucumbers," *Whole Foods*, South Plainfield, N.J., 10:95:68.

Shaw, D. "Duract Pain-Pill Sales are Halted," *Philadelphia Inquirer*, Section C, 6:23:98, pp. C1-C2.

"Shark Cartilage: How It May Take A Bite Out of Cancer," *Whole Foods*, South Plainfield, N.J., 9:95:82.

"Shark Cartilage—The Wellness Breakthrough of the Decade," *Health Food Business*, Melville, N.Y., 9:95:82.

Shealy, C.N., *DHEA, The Youth Hormone*. New Canaan, Conn.:Keats Publishing, 1996.

Shelton, H. *Food Combining Made Easy*. San Antonio, Texas: Willow Publishing, 1994.

Shemo, C.C. "Aromatherapy, The Healing Power of Flowers," *Great Life*, Stamford, Conn., 2:98:20.

Singh, G.B. and C.K. Atal. "Pharmacology of an extract of salai guggal ex-Boswellia Serrata, a new non-steroidal anti-inflammatory agent." *Agents in Action*, 1986, 18:47-12.

Smythe, H. "Tender Points: Evolution of Concepts of the Fibrositis-Fibromyalgia Syndrome," *Amercian Journal of Medicine*, 81 (Supp. 3A) 1986, pp. 2-6.

Sobel, D. and A. C. Klein *Arthritis: What Works*. New York: St. Martin's Press, 1989.

Social Affairs Unit, Manhattan Institute *Health, Lifestyle, and Environment, Countering the Panic*. New York, 1991, pp. 7-9.

Srimal, R. and Dhawn, B. "Pharmacology of Diferuloylo Methane (curcumin); a Non-Steriodal Anti-Inflammatory Agent," *Journal of Pharm. Pharmac.*, 25:447-452, 1973.

Starr, C. and R. Taggart *Biology: The Unity and Diversity of Life*. Belmont, Calif.: Wadsworth Publishing Co., 1987.

Steinberg, D., et al. "Beyond Cholesterol: Modifications of low-density lipoprotein that increase its atherogenicity." *New England Journal of Medicine*, 320:915-24, 1991.

Steinberg, P.N. *Isoflavones and the New Concentrated Soy Supplements*. New York: Healing Wisdom Publications, 1996.

Tappel, A.L. "Selenium Glutathione Peroxidase and Vitamin E," *American Journal of Clinical Nutrition*, (Sept. 1974): 27-960-965.

Theodosakis, J., et al. *The Arthritis Cure*. New York: St. Martin's Press, 1997.

Thorpe, K.E. "How Americans Perceive the Health Care System," *National Coalition on Health Care*, Washington, DC, 1:97.

Tkac, D. "Gout, Coping Ideas" In: *The Doctor's Book of Home Remedies*. (Editors of *Prevention Magazine*), Emmaus, Pa.: Rodale Press, 1990, pp. 309-313.

"Turmeric (Curcuma Longa)," *Let's Live*, Los Angeles, Calif., 12:97:10.

Twickenham, D.W., "Calcium Pantothenate in Arthritic Conditions," Report No. 199 of the General Practitioner Research Group, *Practitioner*, February, 1980, 224: 208-211.

Vaz, A.L. "Double-Blind Clinical Evaluation of the Relative Efficacy of Ibuprofen and Glucosamine Sulfate in the Management of Osteoarthritis of the Knee in out-patients." *Curr. Med. Res Opin.* 8: 145-9, 1982.

"Vitamin E Consumption on the Rise," *The Vitamin Retailer*, New Brunswick, N.J., 4:98:20.

Wade, C. *Vitamin E, The Rejuvenation Vitamin*. New York: Ace Books, 1970.

Wade, C. *Health from the Hive*. New Canaan, Conn.: Keats Publishing, 1992.

Walker, M. "Alpha Lipoic Acid, Total Cell Protection," *Health Food Business*, Melville, N.Y., 1:98:100.

Walker, M. "Bovine Tracheal Cartilage," *Health Food Business*, Melville, N.Y., 2:95:21.

Walker, M. "Kombucha: New Interest in Ancient Culture," *Health Food Business*, Howmark, N.J., 2:96:34.

Walker, M. "Nutritional Medicine, Curcuminoids," *Health Food Business*, Howmark, N.J., 3:98:56.

Walker, N.W. *Fresh Vegetable and Fruit Juices*. Prescott, Ariz.: Norwalk Press, 1970.

Warmbrand, M. *The Encyclopedia of Health and Nutrition*. New York: Pyramid Books, 1962.

Waterson, R.P. "Arthritis: Biochemical Suffocation," *Southwestern Medicine*, Vol. 42, No. 4, April, 1961.

Wei, H., et al. "Antioxidant and Anti-Promotional Effects of the Soy Bean Isoflavone Genistein," *Proceedings of the Society for Experimental Biology and Medicine*, 208(1):124-30, 1:95.

Weil, A. *8 Weeks to Optimum Health*. New York: Alfred A. Knopf, 1997.

Weil, A. *Health and Healing*, New York: Houghton Mifflin Co., 1995.

Weil, A. *Spontaneous Healing*, New York: Alfred A. Knopf, Inc., 1995.

Weiner, M. *More Precious Than Gold: Enzymes*. Toronto, Ontario: GeroVita Laboratories, 1996.

Whitaker, J. *Dr. Whitaker's Guide to Natural Healing*. Rocklin, Calif.: Prima Publishing, 1995.

Williams, R. J. *Nutrition Against Disease* New York: Pitman Publishing, 1985.

Williamson, M.E. *Fibro-Myalgia: A Comprehensive Approach*. New York: Walker and Co., 1996.

Willix, R.D. *You Can Feel Good All the Time*, Baltimore, Md.: Health For Life, 1994.

Wilson, R. "Natural Nutrition, Food Combining. The Missing Link to Better Nutrition," *Let's Live*, Los Angeles, 10:94: 58-60.

Wolfe, A.C.D. *Reclaim Your Inner Terrain*. Wolfe Clinic, Nova Scotia.

Wood, H.C. *Overfed but Undernourished, Nutritional Aspects of Health and Disease*. New York: Exposition Press, 1959.

Young, G. "The PH Factor, The Real Silent Killer," *The Vaxa Journal, The Health Magazine of Prevention and Regeneration*, San Diego, Calif., 1997, p. 3-5.

Zumer, R.B. and M. Ballas "Prostaglandin E suppression of adjuvant Arthritis;" *Arthritis and Rheumatism*, 16 (1973), 251-6.

INDEX

ABOUT THE AUTHOR

George Redmon was born in Edenton, North Carolina and resided most of his life in Philadelphia, Pennsylvania. He graduated with honors and earned his Bachelor's degree in health in 1974. In that same year he was honored as a member of *Who's Who Among College Students In America*.

Dr. Redmon is a graduate of the Clayton School of Natural Healing (N.D.), The American Holistic College of Nutrition, and Walden University (1994) where he earned his Ph.D. He has developed a twenty-year career specializing in holistic healthcare within the vitamin and natural healthcare industry, and has served as a regional and national education director for one of the largest health products companies in the United States. His work has been published in *American Fitness*.

He is a member of the South Jersey Holistic Health Association; the Holistic Health Association of Princeton, New Jersey; the Doctoral Association of New York Educators; Healthier Lifestyles; and the Herbal Healer Academy. Dr. Redmon serves as a consultant to the Center for Stress Pain and Wellness in Wilmington, Delaware; is on the advisory board of the Clayton School of Natural Health; and teaches as an adjunct faculty member with the Washington Township School system in Sewell, New Jersey. He currently resides in Sicklerville, New Jersey with his wife Brenda, and their son George.

Dr. Redmon is the author of *Minerals: Are You Getting Enough?* (Garden City Park, N.Y.: Avery Publishing, 1998).

ADDITIONAL HEALTH TITLES FROM HOHM PRESS

10 ESSENTIAL HERBS, REVISED EDITION
by Lalitha Thomas

Peppermint. . .Garlic. . .Ginger. . .Cayenne. . .Clove. . . and 5 other everyday herbs win the author's vote as the "Top 10" most versatile and effective herbal applications for hundreds of health and beauty needs. *Ten Essential Herbs* offers fascinating stories and easy, step-by-step direction for both beginners and seasoned herbalists. Learn how to use cayenne for headaches, how to make a facial scrub with ginger, how to calm motion sickness and other stomach distress with peppermint. Special sections in each chapter explain the application of these herbs with children and pets too. **Over 25,000 copies in print.**

Paper, 395 pages, $16.95, ISBN: 0-934252-48-3

• • •

DHEA: THE ULTIMATE REJUVENATING HORMONE
by Hasnain Walji, Ph.D.

A sane approach to the use of this age-slowing hormone. Many studies indicate DHEA's positive usage for athletes and others concerned with losing weight without reducing caloric intake, as an aid to both short and long-term memory loss, and in such conditions as diabetes, cancer, Chronic Fatigue Syndrome, heart disease and immune system deficiencies. Contains a comprehensive but user-friendly review of research and relevant nutritional information.

Paper, 95 pages, $9. 95, ISBN: 0-934252-70-X

• • •

KAVA: Nature's Relaxant For Anxiety, Stress and Pain
by Hasnain Walji, Ph.D.

KAVA is currently one of the hottest products in the natural medicine and health-food trade. This book provides consumers with a readable introduction and a balanced and authoritative treatment. KAVA has been shown to relieve the anxiety, tension and restlessness that characterize STRESS, a major contributing factor in the most deadly diseases of our times.

Paper, 144 pages, $9.95   ISBN: 0-934252-78-5

**TO ORDER PLEASE SEE ACCOMPANYING ORDER FORM
OR CALL 1-800-381-2700 TO PLACE YOUR ORDER NOW.**

ADDITIONAL HEALTH TITLES FROM HOHM PRESS

YOUR BODY CAN TALK: How to Use Simple Muscle Testing to Listen to What Your Body Knows and Needs
by Susan L. Levy, D.C. and Carol Lehr, M.A.

Clear instructions in **simple muscle testing**, together with over 25 simple tests for how to use it for specific problems or disease conditions. Special chapters deal with health problems specific to women (especially PMS and Menopause) and problems specific to men (like stress, heart disease, and prostate difficulties). Contains over 30 diagrams, plus a complete Index and Resource Guide.

Paper, 350 pages, $19.95, ISBN: 0-934252-68-8

• • •

NATURAL HEALING WITH HERBS
by Humbart "Smokey" Santillo, N.D.
Foreword by Robert S. Mendelsohn, M.D.

Dr. Santillo's first book, and Hohm Press' long-standing bestseller, is a classic handbook on herbal and naturopathic treatment. Acclaimed as the most comprehensive work of its kind, *Natural Healing With Herbs* details (in layperson's terms) the properties and uses of 120 of the most common herbs and lists comprehensive therapies for more than 140 common ailments. All in alphabetical order for quick reference.

Over 150,000 copies in print.
Paper, 408 pages, $16.95, ISBN: 0-934252-08-4

• • •

10 ESSENTIAL FOODS
by Lalitha Thomas

Carrots, broccoli, almonds, grapefruit and six other miracle foods will enhance your health when used regularly and wisely. Lalitha gives in-depth nutritional information plus flamboyant and good-humored stories about these foods, based on her years of health and nutrition counseling. Each chapter contains easy and delicious recipes, tips for feeding kids and helpful hints for managing your food dollar. A bonus section supports the use of 10 Essential Snacks.

Paper, 300 pages, $16.95, ISBN: 0-934252-74-2

TO ORDER PLEASE SEE ACCOMPANYING ORDER FORM OR CALL 1-800-381-2700 TO PLACE YOUR ORDER NOW.

ADDITIONAL HEALTH TITLES FROM HOHM PRESS

FOOD ENZYMES: THE MISSING LINK TO RADIANT HEALTH
by Humbart "Smokey" Santillo, N.D.

Santillo's breakthrough book presents the most current research in this field, and encourages simple, straightforward steps for how to make enzyme supplementation a natural addition to a nutrition-conscious lifestyle. Special sections on: • Longevity and disease • The value of raw food and juicing • Detoxification • Prevention of allergies and candida • Sports and nutrition

Over 200,000 copies in print.
Paper, 108 pages, U.S. $7.95, ISBN: 0-934252-40-8 (English)
Paper, 108 pages, U.S. $6.95, ISBN: 0-934252-49-1 (Spanish)

■ Audio version of Food Enzymes
2 cassette tapes, 150 minutes, U.S. $17.95, ISBN: 0-934252-29-7

• • •

INTUITIVE EATING: EveryBody's Guide to Vibrant Health and Lifelong Vitality Through Food
by Humbart "Smokey" Santillo, N.D.

The natural voice of the body has been drowned out by the shouts of addictions, over-consumption, and devitalized and preserved foods. Millions battle the scale daily, experimenting with diets and nutritional programs, only to find their victories short-lived at best, confusing and demoralizing at worst. *Intuitive Eating* offers an alternative—a tested method for: • strengthening the immune system • natural weight loss • increasing energy • making the transition from a degenerative diet to a regenerative diet • slowing the aging process.

Paper, 450 pages, $16.95, ISBN: 0-934252-27-0

• • •

THE MELATONIN AND AGING SOURCEBOOK
by Dr. Roman Rozencwaig, M.D. and Dr. Hasnain Walji, Ph.D.

This book covers the latest research on the pineal...control of aging, melatonin and sleep, melatonin and immunity, melatonin's role in cancer treatment, antioxidant qualities of melatonin, dosages, counter indications, quality control, and use with other drugs, melatonin application to heart disease, Alzheimer's, diabetes, stress, major depression, seasonal affective disorders, AIDS, SIDS, cataracts, autism...and many other conditions.

Cloth, 220 pages, $79.95, ISBN: 0-934252-73-4

TO ORDER PLEASE SEE ACCOMPANYING ORDER FORM OR CALL 1-800-381-2700 TO PLACE YOUR ORDER NOW.

ADDITIONAL HEALTH TITLES FROM HOHM PRESS

MANAGING AND PREVENTING ARTHRITIS
The Natural Alternatives
by George L. Redmon, N.D., Ph.D.

Discover a full range of natural alternatives for the prevention of arthritis and other arthritic disturbances, such as gout and fibromyalgia; for slowing the progress of existing arthritis, and for relief of the pain, swelling and stiffness of this disease.

   Learn about dietary change as the major form of prevention; the essential role of antioxidants, vitamins and minerals; the use of herbal treatments; revolutionary supplements, such as glucosamaine sulfate; and the irreplaceable role of positive attitude and self-responsibility in managing, treating and preventing arthritis.

Paper, 182 pages, $12.95, ISBN: 0-934252-90-1

• • •

A VEGETARIAN DOCTOR SPEAKS OUT
by Charles Attwood, M.D., F.A.A.P.
By the famed author of *Dr. Attwood's Low-Fat Prescription for Kids* (Viking, 1995), this new book proclaims the life-saving benefits of a plant-based diet. Twenty-six powerful essays speak out against the myths, the prejudices and the ignorance surrounding the subject of nutrition in the U.S. today. Read about the link between high-fat consumption and heart disease, cancer and other killers; the natural and non-dairy way to increase calcium intake; obesity and our children—more than a matter of genes!; controlling food allergies, for the rest of your life, and many more topics of interest and necessity.

Paper, 167 pages, $14.95, ISBN: 0-934252-85-8

• • •

■ *HERBS, NUTRITION AND HEALING ;* AUDIO CASSETTE SERIES
by Dr. Humbart "Smokey" Santillo, N.D.

Santillo's most comprehensive seminar series. Topics covered in-depth include: • the history of herbology • specific preparation of herbs for tinctures, salves, concentrates, etc. • herbal dosages in both acute and chronic illnesses • use of cleansing and transition diets • treating colds and flu... and more.

4 cassettes, 330 minutes, $40.00, ISBN: 0-934252-22-X

TO ORDER PLEASE SEE ACCOMPANYING ORDER FORM OR CALL 1-800-381-2700 TO PLACE YOUR ORDER NOW.

ADDITIONAL HEALTH TITLES FROM HOHM PRESS

■ *NATURE HEALS FROM WITHIN;* AUDIO CASSETTE SERIES
by Dr. Humbart "Smokey" Santillo, N.D.

Topics include: • The innate wisdom of the body. • The essential role of elimination and detoxification • Improving digestion • How "transition dieting" will take off the weight—for good! • The role of heredity, diet, and prevention in health • How to overcome tiredness, improve your immune system and live longer...and happier.

1 cassette, $8.95, ISBN: 0-934252-66-1

• • •

■ *LIVE SEMINAR ON FOOD ENZYMES*; AUDIO CASSETTE SERIES
by Dr. Humbart "Smokey" Santillo, N.D.

An in-depth discussion of the properties of food enzymes, describing their valuable use to maintain vitality, immunity, health and longevity. Complements all the information in the book.

1 cassette, $8.95, ISBN: 0-934252-29-7

• • •

■ *FRUITS AND VEGETABLES—The Basis of Health*; AUDIO CASSETTE SERIES
by Dr. Humbart "Smokey" Santillo, N.D.

Explains the essential difference between a live food diet, which heals the body, and degenerative foods, which weaken the immune system and cause disease. Recipes included.

1 cassette, $8.95, ISBN: 0-934252-65-3

• • •

■ *WEIGHT-LOSS SEMINAR*; AUDIO CASSETTE SERIES
by Dr. Humbart "Smokey" Santillo, N.D.

This seminar explains the worthlessness of most dietary regimens and explodes many common myths about weight gain. Santillo stresses: • The essential distinction between "good" fats and "bad" fats • The necessity for protein and how to use it efficiently • How to get our primary vitamins and minerals from food • How to ease into becoming an "intuitive eater."

1 cassette, $8.95, ISBN: 0-934252-75-0

TO ORDER PLEASE SEE ACCOMPANYING ORDER FORM OR CALL 1-800-381-2700 TO PLACE YOUR ORDER NOW.

RETAIL ORDER FORM FOR HOHM PRESS HEALTH BOOKS

Name_____ Phone ( )_____

Street Address or P.O. Box _____

City _____ State _____ Zip Code _____

	QTY	TITLE	ITEM PRICE	TOTAL PRICE	
1		**10 ESSENTIAL FOODS**	$16.95		
2		**10 ESSENTIAL HERBS**	$16.95		
3		**MANAGING AND PREVENTING ARTHRITIS**	$12.95		
4		**DHEA: The Ultimate Rejuvenating Hormone**	$9.95		
5		**FOOD ENZYMES/ENGLISH**	$7.95		
6		**FOOD ENZYMES/SPANISH**	$6.95		
7		**FOOD ENZYMES BOOK/AUDIO**	$17.95		
8		**FRUITS & VEGETABLES/AUDIO**	$8.95		
9		**HERBS, NUTRITION AND HEALING/AUDIO**	$40.00		
10		**INTUITIVE EATING**	$16.95		
11		**LIVE SEMINAR ON FOOD ENZYMES/AUDIO**	$8.95		
12		**THE MELATONIN AND AGING SOURCEBOOK**	$79.95		
13		**NATURAL HEALING WITH HERBS**	$16.95		
14		**NATURE HEALS FROM WITHIN/AUDIO**	$8.95		
15		**A VEGETARIAN DOCTOR SPEAKS OUT**	$14.95		
16		**WEIGHT LOSS SEMINAR/AUDIO**	$8.95		
17		**YOUR BODY CAN TALK: How to Listen...**	$19.95		

SURFACE SHIPPING CHARGES

1st book $4.00
Each additional item $1.00

SUBTOTAL:
SHIPPING: (see below)
TOTAL:

SHIP MY ORDER

☐ Surface U.S. Mail—Priority
☐ 2nd-Day Air (Mail + $5.00)
☐ UPS (Mail + $2.00)
☐ Next-Day Air (Mail + $15.00)

METHOD OF PAYMENT:

☐ Check or M.O.   Payable to Hohm Press, P.O. Box 2501, Prescott, AZ 86302
☐ Call 1-800-381-2700 to place your credit card order
☐ Or call 1-520-717-1779 to fax your credit card order
☐ Information for Visa/MasterCard order only:

Card #_____–_____–_____–_____ Expiration Date _____

Visit our Website to view our complete catalog: www.hohmpress.com
ORDER NOW! Call 1-800-381-2700 or fax your order to 1-520-717-1779.
(Remember to include your credit card information.)